Defeat
Joint Pains

Includes...

Arthritis • Gout • Tendinitis • Sprains and Strains
Bursitis • Tennis Elbow • Carpel Tunnel Syndrome
Dislocation • Bunions

and their...

Causes • Symptoms • Lab Investigations • Prevention

By

Dr Ritu Jain

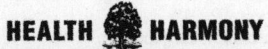

An imprint of

B. Jain Publishers (P) Ltd.
USA — Europe — India

DEFEAT JOINT PAINS

First Edition: 2006
Revised 2nd Edition: 2013
5th Impression: 2013

All rights reserved. No part of this book may be reproduced, stored in a retrieval system or transmitted, in any form or by any means, mechanical, photocopying, recording or otherwise, without any prior written permission of the publisher.

© with the publishers

Published by Kuldeep Jain for

HEALTH 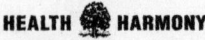 HARMONY
An imprint of
B. JAIN PUBLISHERS (P) LTD.
1921/10, Chuna Mandi, Paharganj, New Delhi 110 055 (INDIA)
Tel.: 91-11-4567 1000 • *Fax:* 91-11-4567 1010
Email: info@bjain.com • *Website:* **www.bjain.com**

Printed in India by
JJ Imprints Pvt. Ltd.

ISBN: 978-81-319-0522-7

Dedication

This book is dedicated

to my parents

Mrs. Malti Shrivastava

and

Mr. Pramod Kumar Shrivastava

Contents

Dedication .... *iii*
Preface .... *xiii*
Acknowledgements .... *xvii*
Publisher's Note .... *xix*
References .... *xxi*

Chapter 1   **What are Joints?** 1
Chapter 2   **Sprains and Strains** 5
- Causes 5
- Symptoms 6
- Lab Investigations 7
- Consult a Doctor if 7
- Treatment and Management 7
  — General 7
  — **Homoeopathy** 8
    - Arnica Montana 30 8
    - Rhus Toxicodendron 30 10
    - Ruta Graveolens 30 12

- ■ Magnesia Phosphorica 30 14
- ■ Calcarea Phosphorica 30 15
- ■ Cinchona Officinalis 30 17
- ■ Strontia Carbonicum 30 19
- — Home Remedies 20
- • Prevention 20

Chapter 3 **Arthritis** **21**
- • Causes 21
- • Types of Arthritis 22
  - — Rheumatoid Arthritis 22
  - — Juvenile Rheumatoid Arthritis 22
  - — Infectious Arthritis 23
  - — Osteoarthritis 23
- • Symptoms 26
- • Lab Investigations 27
  - — Rheumatoid Arthritis 27
  - — Infectious Arthritis 27
  - — Osteoarthritis 27
- • Consult a Doctor if 27
- • Treatment and Management 28
  - — **Homoeopathy** 28
    - ■ Bryonia Alba 30 28
    - ■ Rhus Toxicodendron 30 30
    - ■ Ledum Palustre 30 31
    - ■ Colchicum 30 33
    - ■ Causticum 30 35
    - ■ Magnesia Phosphorica 30 37
    - ■ Pulsatilla 30 39
    - ■ Aconite Napellus 30 41
    - ■ Arnica Montana 30 43
    - ■ Calcarea Phosphorica 30 45
    - ■ Kali Iodide 47
    - ■ Guaiacum ϕ 48

- Rhododendron 30 49
- Kalmia Latifolia 30 51
- Chelidonium Majus 30 52
- Formica Ruta 54
- Lycopodium 30 55
- Sulphur 30 57
- Arsenicum Album 30 60
- Silica 30 62
- Phytolacca 30 64
- Stellaria Medica 30 66
- Mercurius Solubilis 30 67
- Actea Spicata 30 69
- Belladonna 30 70
- Cinchona Officinalis 30 72
- Acid Benzoicum 30 74
- Caulophyllum 30 75

— Acupressure 76
— Herbal Therapy 77
— Hydrotherapy 77
— Yoga 78
— Diet and Nutrition 81
  - What to Eat 81
  - What to Reduce 82
  - What to Avoid 82
— Juice Therapy 82
— Home Remedies 83

Chapter 4 Gout 85
- Causes 86
- Symptoms 87
- Lab Investigations 90
- Consult a Doctor if 90
- Treatment and Management 90
  — **Homoeopathy** 91

- Ledum Palustre 30 91
- Bryonia Alba 30 93
- Acid Benzoicum 30 95
- Lithium Carbonicum 30 96
- Colchicum 30 97
- Lycopodium 30 99
- Mercurius Solubilis 30 101
- Arnica Montana 30 103
- Calcarea Carbonica 30 105
- Causticum 30 107
- Sulphur 30 110
- Rhus Toxicodendron 30 112
- Calcarea Phosphorica 30 114
- Formica Ruta 30 116
- Pulsatilla 30 117
- Staphysagria 30 119
- Aconite Napellus 30 121
- Chinchona Officinalis 30 123
- Guaiacum ϕ 125
- Magnesia Phosphorica 30 126
- Caulophyllum 30 128
— Acupressure 129
— Herbal Therapy 131
— Diet and Nutrition 131
- What to Eat 131
- What to Reduce 131
- What to Avoid 132
— Juice Therapy 132
— Reflexology 133
— Home Remedies 133
• Prevention 134

Chapter 5 **Bursitis 135**
• Causes 136

- Symptoms 136
- Consult a Doctor if 137
- Treatment and Management 137
  - **Homoeopathy** 137
    - Arnica Montana 30 137
    - Phytolacca 30 140
    - Silica 30 141
    - Ruta Graveolens 30 144
    - Rhus Toxicodendron 30 146
    - Acid Benzoicum 30 147
    - Sulphur 30 148
    - Calcarea Phosphorica 30 151
    - Causticum 30 152
    - Bryonica Alba 30 155
    - Kali Iodide 30 157
    - Mercurius Solubilis 30 158
    - Belladonna 30 160
  - Acupressure 162
  - Herbal Therapy 162
  - Juice Therapy 162
  - Bach Flower Therapy 163
  - Diet and Nutrition 163
- Prevention 163

Chapter 6 Tennis Elbow 165
- Causes 167
- Symptoms 167
- Consult a Doctor if 167
- Treatment and Management 168
  - **Homoeopathy** 168
    - Rhus Toxicodendron 30 168
    - Ruta Graveolens 30 170
    - Magnesia Phosphorica 30 172
    - Causticum 30 173

- ■ Pulsatilla 30 176
- ■ Arnica Montana 30 178
- ■ Silica 30 180
— Acupressure 183
— Physiotherapy 183
— Herbal Therapy 184
— Hydrotherapy 184
— Home Remedies 184
• Prevention 185
— Preventing a Tennis Elbow 185
— Preventing Relapse 185

Chapter 7 **Carpal Tunnel Syndrome** **187**
- Causes 189
- Symptoms 190
- Consult a Doctor if 190
- Lab Investigations 191
- Treatment and Management 191
    — **Homoeopathy** 192
    - ■ Pulsatilla 30 192
    - ■ Rhus Toxicodendron 30 194
    - ■ Ruta Graveolens 30 196
    - ■ Arnica Montana 30 198
    - ■ Calcarea Carbonica 30 200
    - ■ Calcarea Phosphorica 30 202
    - ■ Causticum 30 204
    - ■ Lycopodium 207
    - ■ Rhododendron 30 209
    — Acupressure 210
    — Physiotherapy 210
    — Yoga 211
    — Herbal Therapy 211
    — Diet and Nutrition 211
    — Juice Therapy 211

	— Home Remedies	212
	• Prevention	212
Chapter 8	**Tendinitis**	**213**
	• Causes	214
	• Symptoms	214
	• Consult a Doctor if.	215
	• Lab Investigations	215
	• Treatment and Management	215
	— **Homoeopathy**	215
	■ Rhus Toxicodendron 30	216
	■ Phytolacca 30	217
	■ Rhododendron 30	219
	■ Bryonia Alba 30	220
	■ Bellodonna 30	222
	— Physiotherapy	225
	— Herbal Therapy	225
	— Home Remedies	225
	• Prevention	226
Chapter 9	**Dislocation**	**227**
	• Causes	227
	• Symptoms	229
	• Consult a Doctor if.	229
	• Lab Investigations	229
	• Treatment and Management	229
	— **Homoeopathy**	230
	■ Calcarea Carbonica 30	230
	■ Causticum 30	232
	■ Arnica Montana 30	235
	■ Rhus Toxidendron 30	237
	■ Belladonna 30	238
	■ Bryonia Alba 30	241
	■ Ruta Graveolens 30	242
	■ Pulsatilla 30	244

- Kali Iodide 246
- Sulphur 30 248

Chapter 10 Bunions 251
- Causes 252
- Symptoms 252
- Consult a Doctor if 253
- Lab Investigations 253
- Treatment and Management 253
  — **Homoeopathy** 253
    - Silica 30 253
    - Calcarea Carbonica 30 255
    - Acid Benzoicum 30 258
    - Kali Iodide 30 259
    - Rhododendron 30 260
    - Sulphur 30 262
  — Home Remedies 264
- Prevention 265

Preface

My purpose in writing this series of books is to provide the general public information on homoeopathy as well as on some other alternative therapies and their uses in particular health disorders like joint pains, asthma, diabetes, high blood pressure, back pain, constipation etc.

People now wish to take more responsibility for their own health. An increasing number want to understand what they can do themselves to prevent illness and, if they do become ill, to understand the causes and determine how they can help themselves recover. Homoeopathy offers a simple, effective, extremely safe, and relatively inexpensive way of accomplishing this—provided it is practiced with common sense.

By understanding the basics of homoeopathy you will be able to take better care of your physical, mental and emotional well-being. In the market, thousands of homoeopathic remedies are available. This book aims to clear the mysteries surrounding homoeopathy and will help you to make an informed choice about homoeopathic self-treatment.

It is my kind request that under no circumstances, however, should patients suffering from serious ailments (or those uncertain of their ailment) consider self-treatment. They should always consult a well-qualified experienced homoeopathic physician.

Defeat Joint Pains with Homoeopathy & others Alternative Therapies is a practical, jargon-free book for all those who are suffering form joint pains and are taking allopathic painkillers, steroids etc. and getting temporary relief with no cure in sight. Moreover, constant use of allopathic medicines causes numerous side-effects which include damage to the liver, kidneys, heart and reduced immunity. This book will help these people to understand the cause and nature of their joint pains and then make them aware about specific homoeopathic remedies as well as other alternative therapies including yoga, acupressure, diet & nutrition which will help them recover rapidly and permanently.

Highlights of the book are as follows:

✦ Information on homoeopathy—All the questions that you always wanted to ask have been answered. This will help you understand the basics of homoeopathy and integrate it into your healthcare

✦ Many figures, diagrams and illustrations have been included to make the topic interesting and easy to understand

✦ Various types of joints and their structure and functions have been properly explained

- All disorders which cause joint pains have been covered:
  - Sprains & Strains
  - Arthritis—Rheumatoid arthritis, Juvenile rheumatoid arthritis, Infectious arthritis, Osteoarthritis
  - Gout
  - Bursitis
  - Tennis Elbow
  - Carpel Tunnel Syndrome
  - Tendinitis
  - Dislocation
  - Bunions
- Every aspect of each disorder has been explained in easy-to-understand language—Causes, Symptoms, Lab investigations, when to consult a doctor, Treatment and management & Prevention
- Under homoeopathic treatment, only those remedies which have been found very effective in a particular disorder have been listed with their indicated symptoms and dosages. This makes the choice of remedy very effortless
- In addition to homoeopathic treatment, the following complementary therapies have been included:
  - Bach flower therapy
  - Home remedies
  - Acupressure
  - Reflexology
  - Herbal therapy
  - Hydrotherapy

- Yoga
- Diet & nutrition
- Juice therapy
- Massage
- Exercises
- Physiotherapy

✦ With the help of the above-mentioned additional information the patient can complement the homoeopathic treatment with other suitable therapies to get maximum benefit in the shortest time

Above all else, as you work your way through this book, keep in mind a message of hope. Whether your disorder is recent or lifelong, you are walking a road taken by many others. They are still travelling, but the road is getting easier as they move ahead rather than stand still. From this book you will learn treatments that are based on research, evidence and experience. They work— and they will work for you. All the best with your journey. Now it is time to begin . . .

Dr Ritu Jain

Acknowledgements

I would never have started writing this book if Dr Rohit Jain, my husband who is also Publishing Manager with B. Jain Publishers, had not invited me to do so and then encouraged and supported me along the way—thanks, Rohit. Also how can I forget my lovely 1 year-old daughter Adya who kept me refreshed with her innocent activities.

My indebtedness to Dr Vijay Kansal and Dr Shailendra Shrivastava, both are Orthopedic Consultants, for their constant help and motivation. I am also thankful to Dr Vimal K. Bhardwaj for beautifully drawing the diagrams of the book.

My thanks also to my publisher, Mr Kuldeep Jain, who approached me to put my knowledge together and form this book—and then helped me!

I am sincerely grateful to my patients who have enriched my experience and confidence over the years. And to my brother, sisters, their families, and my friends for their inspiration and support.

Publisher's Note

History bears testimony to the fact that life in the early times was not stressful like today. The life span of mankind was much longer and devoid of many ailments.

But with the passage of time and the advancement of technology, man has progressed though at the cost of many things, especially their health. Man's life today is replete with worries and health problems. When such is the scenario, then man thinks of getting cured easily as time is a big factor and also thinks of preventions to check illnesses.

At such a juncture comes this excellent book of Dr Ritu Jain which talks about various kinds of joint related diseases, their management and also prevention. She has effectively given guidance regarding the usage of homeopathic medicines and also how to control these diseases through alternative therapies as allopathic medicines sometimes harm the patients.

We are extremely pleased to publish this book and we hope many people suffering from different types of joint pains will benefit from it

Kuldeep Jain
CEO, B. Jain Publishers (P) Ltd.

References

While no reference has been made to authors through the work owing to the writer's desire to economize space, yet she desires to express her indebtedness to the numerous writers upon these subjects as they have each been freely consulted in the preparation of this work.

CHAPTER 1

What are Joints?

Adjacent bones are joined by ligaments and the strong fibrous capsule that surrounds the joint. Joint cavity is covered by synovial membrane. Synovial membrane produces a lubricating fluid. Within a joint, adjacent bone surfaces are covered with hyaline cartilage. Hyaline cartilage is a hard clear ultra smooth material. Especially strong, shock-absorbing cartilage is found in the knee joint and the disc between the vertebrae. *(See figure 1.1)*

Joints between few bones are fixed, for examples in the skull. Other joints allow a variety of movement like girding, pivoting, rotating and hinge action. The elbow joint is a hinge joint, shown in figure *1.2 (a)*. The ball-socket joint at the shoulder & hip joints allows bending & rotation through a number of different planes, as shown in figure *1.2 (b)*. The joints between the vertebrae act like a flexible washer, allowing the spine to turn & bend, as shown in figure *1.2 (c)*.

Joint Pain

Pain in joints could be due to various ailments & problems. Read down this page to find out the various possibilities:

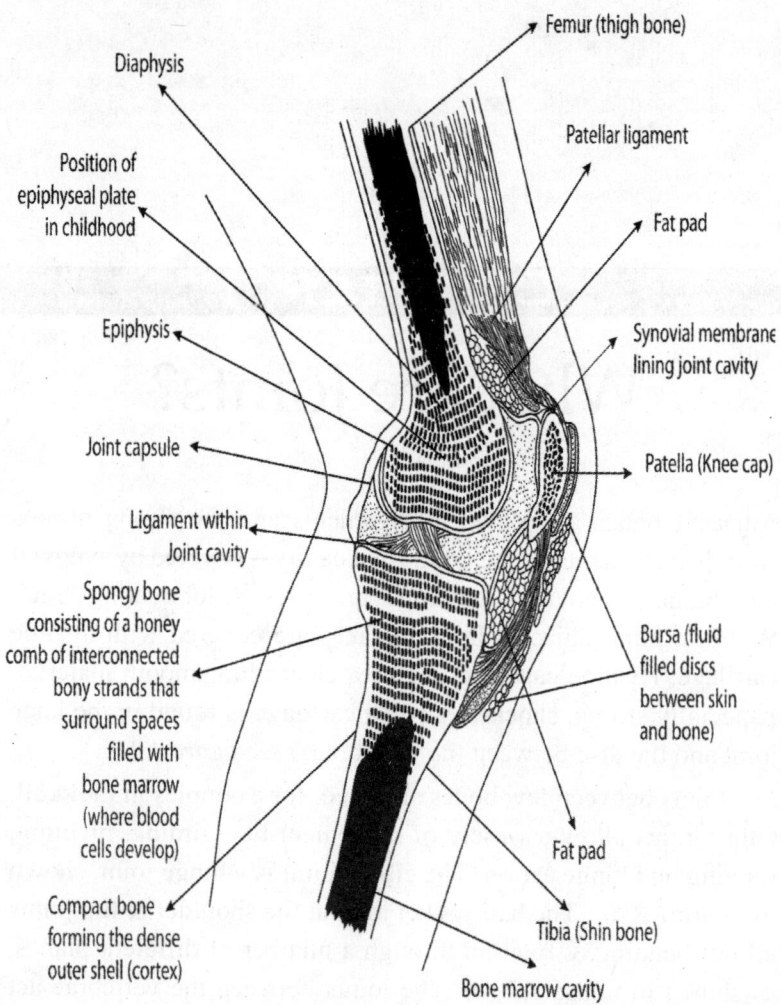

Fig. 1.1 *Knee Joint*

What are Joints?

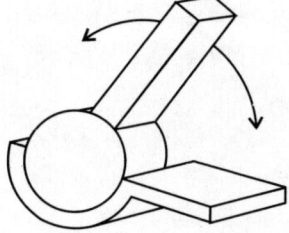 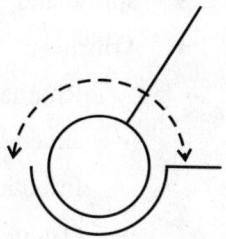

(a) Hinge Joint; Example Elbow Joint

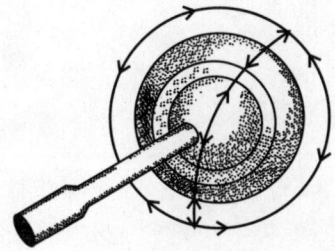 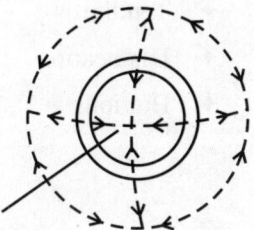

*(b) Ball & Socket Joint Allows Bending and Rotation;
Example Shoulder and Hip Joint*

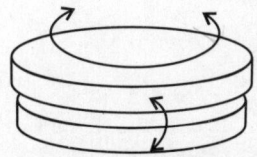 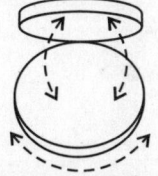

(c) Vertebral Joint Allowing the Spine to Turn and Bend

Fig. 1.2 *Degrees of Bending, Rotation or Both,
Allowed by Such a Joint*

- Sprain and Strain
- Arthritis
  - Rhumatonid arthritis
  - Juvenile rheumotoid arthritis
  - Infectious arthritis
  - Osteoarthritis
- Gout
- Bursitis
- Tennis Elbow
- Carpal Tunnel Syndrome
- Tendinitis
- Dislocation
- Bunions

Chapter 2

Sprains and Strains

Sprains and Strains are the most common form of injury and range from twisting of ankle to aching backs.

A *Sprain* injures the ligaments which are the tough, fibrous bands of tissue that connect the bones to one another at a joint. (See figure 2.1)

A *Strain* damages muscle and tendons that attach muscle to the bone. The tendon gets stretched or torn.

Causes

- Sudden or unaccustomed stress on joint or muscle
- Falls
- Lifting heavy objects
- Playing unfamiliar sports

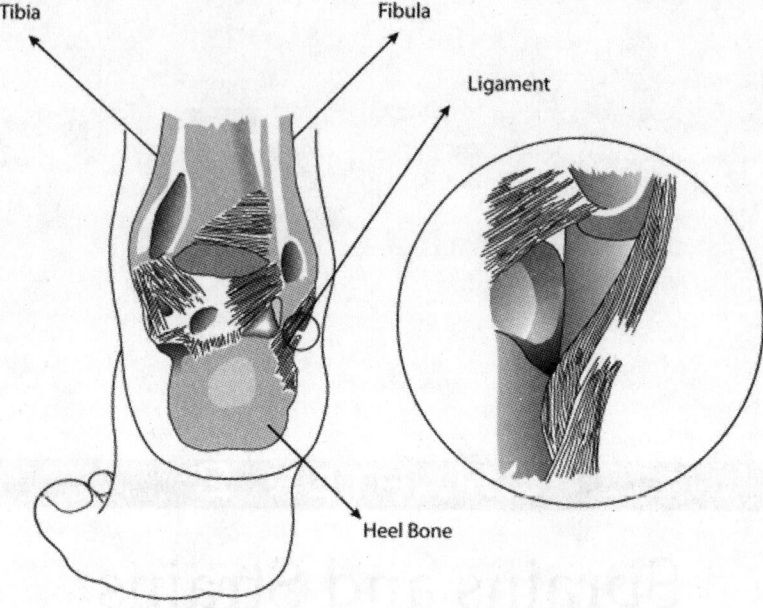

Fig. 2.1 *Sprained Ankle Joint—The Ligaments are Stretched and Torn*

✦ Being obese, inactive or having poor physical health increases the chances of sprains and strains

Symptoms
Sprains... • Pain in the injured joint • Rapid swelling of the joint, mostly with bruising • Stiffness and difficulty in moving the joint ***Strains...*** • Sharp pain at the site of injury • Pain is followed by stiffness, tenderness and swelling

Lab Investigations

- ✦ X-rays to rule out fracture
- ✦ MRI scan is done to find out ruptured tissues

Consult a Doctor if

- ✦ The pain, swelling and stiffness does not improve within three days
- ✦ There is a popping sensation when you move the injured joint
- ✦ There is inability to move the injured joint; this may be due to fracture
- ✦ There are repeated sprains and strains

Treatment and Management

Treatment aims to control the pain and swelling, followed by rest which allows healing. Most sprains and strains heal within 2-3 weeks.

General . . .

Treatment in the first 24 hours : **'RICE'**.

Rest: Rest to the affected area to avoid further injury.

Ice: Apply ice packs alternately. It helps in reducing the swelling and inflammation.

Compression: It restricts the swelling. Use elastic bandage to compress the area and reduce swelling.

Elevation: Elevate the affected part above the heart to improve drainage from the affected part and to reduce pain.

After 48-72 hrs. you may use hot fomentation to relieve soreness and stimulate circulation of the affected area. Your doctor may advise heat or infrared treatment from a physiotherapist.

Homoeopathy

Massage the area with *Rhus tox. or Arnica* ointment to reduce the soreness and tenderness.

Following remedies are usually indicated in Sprains and Strains:

Arnica Montana 30

4 pills three times daily for one month

Symptoms
- ✦ Rheumatism of muscular and tendinous tissue, especially of hip, back and shoulders
- ✦ It is suited to cases when any injury, however remote, seems to have caused the present trouble
- ✦ A muscular tonic
- ✦ Limbs and body aches as if beaten; joints as if sprained
- ✦ *Sore, lame and bruised feeling*
- ✦ Sharp, shooting, paralytic or sprained pains which quickly change place
- ✦ *Gouty affections.* Great fear at being touched or approached

Symptoms *Worse*
- **Least touch**
- **Motion**
- **Rest**
- **Wine**
- **Damp cold**
- **Evening**
- **From speaking**
- **Blowing nose**
- **Almost any noise**
- **Lying on the injured part**
- **From over-exertion**
- **Alcohol**
- **Old age**

Sprains and Strains

- Sore, tender, red swelling of the joints in gout, particularly of knee joint
- Gout with arthritic pains in the feet and the big toe as if sprained
- In arthritis, especially the hip joint is affected
- Rheumatism begins low down and work up
- Cannot walk erect, on account of bruised pain in pelvic region
- Paralytic pains in all joints during motion
- Knee bends suddenly when walking, stitches when touched
- Twitching pain from left shoulder joint to middle finger
- Pain in back and limbs, as if bruised
- Deathly coldness of forearms
- Everything on which the person lies seems too hard
- Soreness after over-exertion
- Cracking in the right wrist when the hand is moved, as if dislocated
- During *Sprains* and Strains, ligaments torn with swelling is most prominent. Bruising and inflammation of the soft tissue around the joint
- When muscles or soft tissues are black and blue

Symptoms *Better*
• Lying down
• Lying with head low
• Warmth
• Rubbing and wrapping up warmly
• Long walk in cold weather
• Outstretched
• Changing the position

Following symptoms generally accompany the above symptoms...

- Produces conditions similar to those resulting from injuries, falls, blows, contusions
- Especially suited to cases when any injury occurs; *after any traumatic injuries*
- Remote effects of injuries even though received years ago
- Whole body feels sore and bruised, lame and does not want to be approached, touched or jarred
- It *promotes healing*, reduces swelling, prevents pus formation
- It is very effective in any kind of bleeding
- Head hot with cold body
- Fetid breath
- Diarrhoea offensive and bloody
- *Violent spasmodic cough with facial herpes*
- Skin black and blue. Multiple small boils very painful. Acne characterised by *symmetry in distribution*
- *Aids recovery after an operation*

Rhus Toxicodendron 30

4 pills three times daily for one month

Symptoms

- Hot, painful swelling of joint
- Tearing and drawing pain
- *Limbs stiff, paralysed sensation*
- Tenderness about knee joint
- Trembling after exertion
- Tingling in feet

Sprains and Strains

- Loss of power in forearm and fingers
- Crawling sensation in the tips of finger
- Tearing *pain in tendons, ligament and fasciae*
- Numbness and tomification after overwork and exposure
- Soreness of condyles of bones
- Pains aching, sore, bruised, tearing, shooting with heaviness, lameness and stiffness
- *Sprains, strains, torn ligaments and tendinitis*

The following symptoms generally accompany the above symptoms ...

- *Extreme restlessness* accompanies most symptoms. Cannot stay in one position, continued change of position
- Aching in bone with fever
- Tongue coated, except red triangular space at tip with great thirst
- Bitter taste in mouth
- Skin eruptions—red, swollen with intense itching
- Desire for milk
- Fever of typhoid character
- General or localised glandular swelling

Symptoms *Worse*

- The cold fresh air is not tolerable
- Damp weather and after rains
- From sitting and rising from sitting position or first attempt to move
- Approach of storms
- At night, especially in bed
- After overwork and exposure
- From gardening
- Checked perspiration
- Injuries after lifting and over exertion

- ✦ Trembling and palpitation of heart when siting still
- ✦ *Sensitive to open air,* putting the hand from under the bed-cover brings on cough

Ruta Graveolens 30
4 pills three times daily for one month

Symptoms
- ✦ It acts upon bone, joints producing symptoms of a rheumatic nature
- ✦ For bruises that occurs on bone, e.g. chin, elbow, skull
- ✦ Pain is felt on the surface of bone, particularly places where tendons are attached to the bone
- ✦ There is bruised pain all over the body, as after a fall, worse in limbs, spine and joints
- ✦ Especially in *sprains and strains* after injury when *Arnica* and *Rhus tox.* do not help
- ✦ Tendon or ligament that have been torn or wrenched
- ✦ Pain feels closer to the bone and can be associated with hard swelling where the tendon is attached to the bone
- ✦ Pain and stiffness in *wrist* and hands
- ✦ Tearing in right wrist, worse with motion; pain in left wrist as it broken
- ✦ Bursa and ganglion of wrist
- ✦ *Veins of hands swell after eating. Fingers distorted*

Symptoms *Better*
• From external heat
• Warm compresses
• From warmth of bed
• Continued movement
• Change of position
• Moving affected part
• Rubbing
• From stretching out limbs

Sprains and Strains

- ✦ Wrenching pain in shoulder joints when the arms are allowed to hang down or when resting on them
- ✦ Pain between scapulae in the afternoon
- ✦ Tension and pressure in shoulders with stiffness in the morning
- ✦ *Thighs pain when stretching the limbs;* on rising from a seat, thighs and hips so weak, they are unable to support body weight so that he falls back on the seat
- ✦ Aching pain in tendo-achilles
- ✦ *Lameness and pain in ankle* with puffy swelling
- ✦ Hamstring feels shortened
- ✦ *Tendons sore;* working leaves patient weary and weak
- ✦ Pain in bones at feet and ankles. Pain in them does not permit to step heavily
- ✦ In *Tennis elbow* pain sore, bruised with lameness, worse from exercise

Symptoms *Worse*
• Lying down especially lying on the painful part
• From cold
• Cold damp weather
• Rest
• Over-excretion
• Sitting or rising from a seat
• Lifting
• On stooping
• Beginning to move

Symptoms *Better*
• Dry warm weather
• Warmth
• Moving about

The following symptoms generally accompany the above symptoms...

- ✦ Feeling of intense lassitude, weakness and despair
- ✦ Restless, changes position frequently when lying

- ✦ All parts of body painful as if bruised
- ✦ Eyes painful with blurred vision from fine work like sewing or reading. Eyes red, hot and painful
- ✦ Difficult stool
- ✦ Even after urination constant urging to urinate, feels bladder full
- ✦ Backache relieved by lying flat on the back

Magnesia Phosphorica 30

4 pills three times daily for one month

Symptoms

- ✦ Neuralgia pain and cramping of muscles
- ✦ In sprain and strain, sharp, stabbing, shooting pain
- ✦ Pain generally sharp, cutting, piercing, knife like, stabbing, shooting, stitching, lightening like
- ✦ Involuntary shaking of hands
- ✦ Cramps in calves
- ✦ Writer's and player's cramp
- ✦ Weakness in arms and legs
- ✦ Finger tips numb and stiff
- ✦ General muscular weakness

Symptoms *Worse*
- On the right side
- Touch
- Night
- Cold bathing or washing
- Being uncovered
- Walking in fresh air

Symptoms *Better*
- Warmth and heat
- Bending double
- Pressure
- Friction

The following symptoms generally accompany the above symptoms . . .

- Suitable for leans thin emaciated persons who are forgetful, easily tired, drowsy, averse to mental effort
- Main remedy for *spasmodic pain; generally sudden and severe*
- Painful ailment relieved by the *application of heat*
- Pain shifts rapidly and usually affects right side of the body
- Craving for sugar, averse to coffee
- May have thirst for cold drinks
- *Menstrual cramping* better after the flow begins
- Indicated for *all forms of cramp,* spasmodic and neuralgic pains in head, face, teeth, abdomen or stomach
- A fine remedy for the tummy pains of babies
- Flatulent colic, forcing the patient to bend double, accompanied with belching of gas, which gives no relief. Bloated abdomen, must loosen the clothes, walk about and constantly pass flatus
- Spasmodic cough, whooping cough
- Angia pectoris
- In fever, chills run up and down the back with shivering
- Great dread of cold air, *of uncovering*, of touching affected part, of cold bathing or walking, of moving

Calcarea Phosphorica 30

4 pills three times daily for one month

Symptoms

- Shooting, tearing and aching type of rheumatic pain in all parts of body especially knees, loins and thumb

- Pain with stiffness, coldness, *numbness and crawling sensation*
- Pain become worse by any change of weather
- Buttocks, back and limbs fall asleep
- Weary when going upstairs. Cannot rise from seat. Staggering like old people when rising from a seat
- Pain in joints and bones excited or increased by every draft of cold damp air
- Rheumatism of cold weather, getting well in spring and the condition returning in autumn

The following symptoms generally accompany the above symptom . . .

- For anaemic persons, especially *anaemic children* who are flabby, have cold extremities and feeble digestion
- Children—*emaciated, unable to stand, and slow in learning to walk*
- Feels complaints more when thinking about them
- Numbness and crawling are characteristic sensations
- Symptoms get worse by wet cold air and every *change of weather*

Symptoms *Worse*
- Exposure to cold and damp weather
- Cold air
- Melting snow
- Changeable weather
- East winds
- Mental exertion
- Dinner
- After a meal, especially juicy fruits
- Motion

Symptoms *Better*
- In summer
- Warm, dry atmosphere
- Lying down
- Rest
- Passing wind

- Headache, *worse near the region of sutures*
- Glandular enlargement—swollen tonsils. *Adenoid growths*
- *Craving for bacon, ham, salted or smoked meat*
- *Much flatulence.* Flatulence temporarily relieved by sour eructations
- Pain in abdomen *at every attempt to eat*
- Diarrhoea from juicy fruits, during dentition *with fetid flatus*
- White discharge in females, *like white of egg*

Cinchona Officinalis 30

4 pills three times daily for one month

Symptoms

- It is more useful in chronic cases of gout and rheumatism
- *Pain in limbs and joints, as if sprained, worse at the slight touch* and better by hard pressure
- Joint swollen and very sensitive with dread of open air
- Drawing and tearing pain in every joint
- Tendency of limbs to go to sleep
- Weakness of joints worse in the morning and when sitting
- Paralytic jerking and tearing in long bones, worse with touch
- Pain in thigh bone as if periosteum had been scraped with a dull knife
- Sensation as if there is a string around the limb
- Great debility, trembling and numb sensation
- Knees give away while walking, worse while ascending stairs
- Hot swelling of right knee with pain extending to thigh and leg

- Aversion to exercise and sensitive to touch
- Chronic synovitis of the knee
- In case of chronic gout when it is mono-articular form and also intervals between attacks
- One hand icy cold and other hand warm

The following symptoms generally accompany the above symptoms . . .

- Ailments *from loss of vital fluids, especially haemorrhages,* excessive lactation, diarrhoea
- Symptoms with *marked periodicity,* return every other day, or regularly in season at the same time
- Rapid general weakness with tendency of sweating from least excretion as well as sleep
- Patient is disobedient, depressed and ready to offend others
- Excessive *sensitivity to light, touch* but relief from hard pressure on painful part
- Throbbing headache, as if the skull would burst
- Excessive flatulence of stomach and bowels, belching gives no relief. Abdomen swollen like a drum with gas

Symptoms *Worse*
- Slightest touch
- After eating
- At night
- Drafts of air
- Every other day
- Prolonged exertion
- Motion
- Loss of vital fluids
- Bending over
- From walking which makes the person dizzy
- From fruits and milk
- From perspiration

Symptoms *Better*
- Bending double
- Hard pressure
- Warmth
- Open air
- Loose clothing
- Lying down

- ✦ Frothy, watery, undigested stool; *painless diarrhoea*
- ✦ Passive haemorrhage from all outlets of the body with dark clotted blood
- ✦ *Intermittent fever worse every other day*, no thirst during heat, great thirst during sweat
- ✦ Anaemia and loss of appetite

Strontia Carbonicum 30
4 pills three times daily for one month

Symptoms
- ✦ Chronic sprains
- ✦ *Chronic* sprains particularly of ankle joint
- ✦ *Sprains of ankle joints with swelling* (or oedema)
- ✦ Rheumatic pains especially in joints
- ✦ Rheumatic pain in right shoulder
- ✦ Rheumatism with diarrhoea
- ✦ Pains make patient faint or sick
- ✦ Feet icy-cold
- ✦ Cramps in calves
- ✦ Cramps in soles
- ✦ Engorged veins of hands
- ✦ Affections of bones, especially femur

Symptoms *Worse*
• Change of weather
• When beginning to move
• Sensitiveness to cold
• **From being quiet**

Symptoms *Better*
• In hot water

The following symptoms generally accompany the above symptoms . . .
- ✦ *Chronic sequelae of haemorrhages,* after operations with much oozing of blood and coldness and prostration

- ✦ For *shock after surgical operations*
- ✦ High blood pressure with flushed face
- ✦ Restlessness at night, smothering feeling
- ✦ Neuritis, great sensitiveness to cold
- ✦ *Vertigo with headache and nausea*
- ✦ Burning and redness of eyes
- ✦ Aversion to meat
- ✦ Craving for bread and beer
- ✦ Eructations after eating
- ✦ Diarrhoea, *worse at night, continuous urging*
- ✦ Skin moist, itching and burning eruption, better in open air
- ✦ Profuse sweating at night

If there is no improvement after one month then please consult a trained homoeopathic practitioner.

Home Remedies

For sprains and strains try a hot vinegar pack. Heat equal part of vinegar and water, then soak a towel for a minute. Apply it to the affected area for five minutes. Remove it, then apply a cold one for five minutes, cover with wool. Repeat it three times.

Prevention

Maintaining good physical health is very important to prevent sprains and strains. Yoga is a time-tested approach to build strong and flexible muscles, ligaments and tendons. If you are overweight, consult your doctor for an appropriate diet and exercise program.

Chapter 3

Arthritis

Nowadays people suffer more from pain in joints than due to any other ailment. And this is due to changes in our lifestyle, our jobs, and leisure activities that have become more sedantary.

Arthritis means inflammation of a joint. Generally, people perceive it as any kind of pain or discomfort related with body movement or general stiffness or pain in the joints.

Causes

- As a result of a disease
- An infection
- Connective tissue disorder
- A genetic defect

- Due to aging process
- Autoimmune disorder

Types of Arthritis

There are many types of arthritis. Here, we only discuss a few common types:

Rheumatoid Arthritis

This is the commonest form of chronic inflammatory joint disease. It is also known as rheumatism or synovitis. It usually affects people over 40 years of age and females are more prone. It affects small and large peripheral joints, with systemic disturbance to other parts of the body, including the heart, lungs, eyes, nerves and muscles. The discomfort of rheumatoid arthritis develops slowly and tends to be most severe on awakening.

Rheumatoid arthritis in older people may cause deformity of hands and feet as muscles weaken, tendons shrink, and the ends of bone become abnormally enlarged.

If the treatment is started at the early stage of disease it gives relief to most people. Generally, symptoms may progress for five years or more, eventually they tend to stabilize or decline the movement of joints. So, permanent disability can be prevented by early treatment.

Juvenile Rheumatoid Arthritis

It is an inflammatory arthritis characterised by persistently negative tests for rheumatoid factor associated with numbers of other common features like chronic fever and anaemia, and secondary effects on the heart, lungs, eyes and nervous system. It commences in childhood before the age of 16 years.

In some cases, juvenile rheumatoid arthritis presents with high fever, pericarditis, mono or poly articular synovitis, with progressive erosion of cartilage. Here, rheumatoid factor is not present in blood. This typical type is called *still's disease*.

In children younger than the age of five, juvenile arthritis attack can last for weeks and recurrence is also possible but symptoms may be less severe. Patients require heavy physical therapy and exercise. Nowadays, permanent damage is rare.

Infectious Arthritis

Infective arthritis can accompany septicemia at any age. It is usually a complication of an injury or another disease. It is less common than arthritic conditions that come on with age. Symptoms have an abrupt onset with severe pain and swelling of a single joint associated with a swinging fever, severe malaise or primary injury.

Large joints (arms and leg joints) are most frequently affected. Generally joint is hot, tender and swollen with marked limitation of movement. The diagnosis may be missed and if left untreated, can result in permanent disability.

Osteoarthritis

It is also known as *arthrosis or degenerative joint disease*. It is not a single disease. Rather it is the end-result of a variety of patterns of joint failure. It is a degenerative and destructive disorder of the hyaline cartilage and adjacent bone of joints. It is the most common form of arthritis, particularly in the elders. In osteoarthritis, the protective cartilage at the end of bones in joints, gradually wears away and the inner bone surfaces become exposed and rub together.

It generally confines to one or only a few joints in majority of patients. The joints most frequently involved are those of the spinal joints, hips and knee joints (weight-bearing joints).

The mechanism of osteoarthritis is generally unknown, but some people have genetic predisposition. *Misuse of steroids can also bring an early onset of disease.* It may be due to trauma, joint mal-alignment, foreign bodies and damaged cartilage from septic arthritis.

The symptoms are gradual in onset; pain and stiffness develops gradually. Pain is usually made worse by exercise, whereas stiffness in the morning or after inactivity improves with movement. As the disease progresses, movement in the affected joint becomes increasingly limited, and tenderness and grating sensation develops and crepitus may be felt on joint movement. Overgrowth of all tissues in and around the joint causes joint enlargement. Associated muscle wasting occurs as the disease progresses, causing increasing instability and joints become more prone to injury. Locking of joint may occur, if bony outgrowth (osteophytes) protrude into the joint cavity.

Other arthritic conditions include ankylosing spondylitis (arthritis of the spine), bone spur (bony growths on the vertebrae or other areas), gout (crystal arthritis), and systemic lupus (inflammatory connective tissue disease).

Arthritis

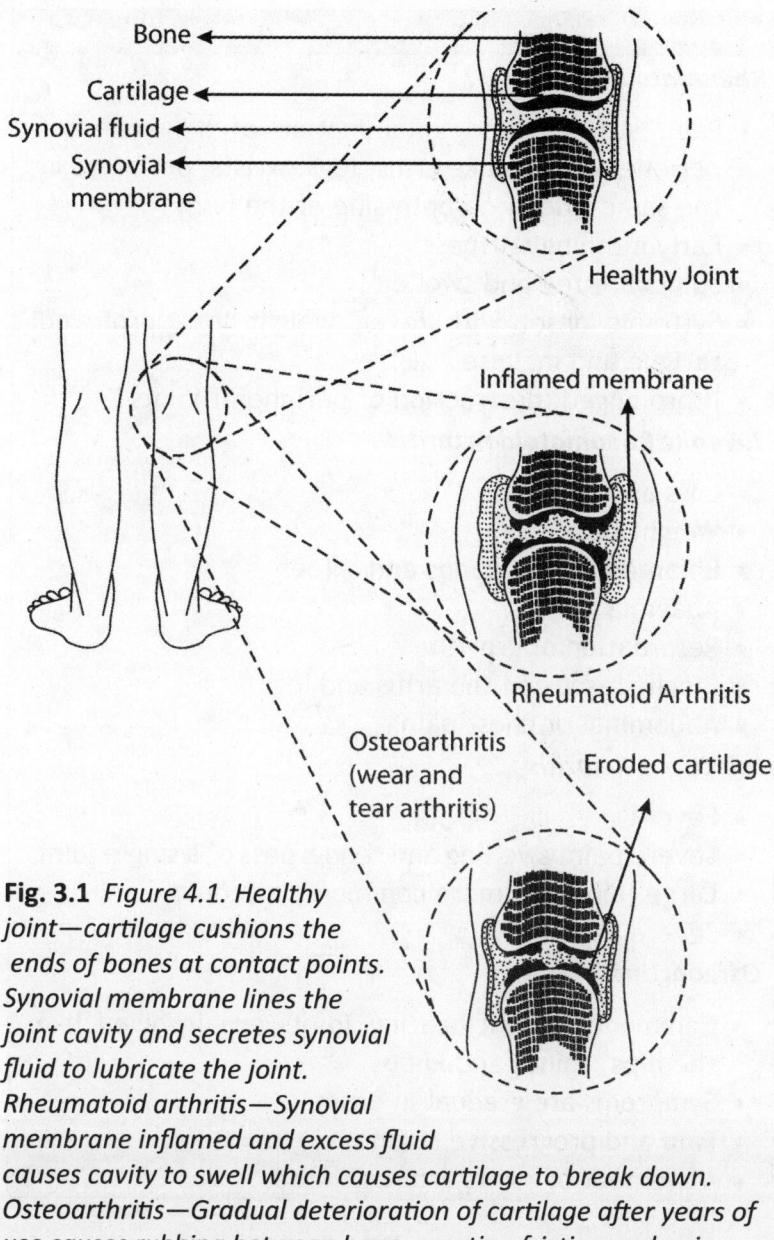

Fig. 3.1 Figure 4.1. Healthy joint—cartilage cushions the ends of bones at contact points. Synovial membrane lines the joint cavity and secretes synovial fluid to lubricate the joint. Rheumatoid arthritis—Synovial membrane inflamed and excess fluid causes cavity to swell which causes cartilage to break down. Osteoarthritis—Gradual deterioration of cartilage after years of use causes rubbing between bone, creating friction and pain

Symptoms

Rheumatoid Arthritis

- Pain, stiffness and inflammation of a number of peripheral joints like arms, legs, wrists, or fingers in the same side or on both side of the body
- Early morning stiffness
- Joints are red and swollen
- Systemic onset with fever, weight loss, profound fatigue and malaise
- If prolonged, destruction of peripheral joints

Juvenile Rheumatoid Arthritis

- Loss of appetite
- Weight loss
- Enlarged lymph glands and spleen
- Anaemia
- Retardation of growth
- Blochy rashes on the arms and legs
- Abdominal or chest pain

Infectious Arthritis

- Fever
- Severe pain, swelling and tenderness of a single joint
- Large joints are more commonly affected
- Severe malaise

Osteoarthritis

- Commonly weight-bearing joints are involved like the hips, spines and knees
- Symptoms are gradual in onset
- Pain and progressive stiffness
- Movement of joints are restricted

Lab Investigations

Rheumatoid Arthritis

- In addition to sign and symptom analysis, blood tests are commonly done to confirm the diagnosis. A majority of sufferers have antibodies called rheumatoid factor (RA factor)
- Investigation shows high CRP. RA Factor
- X-ray findings

Infectious Arthritis

- Testing a sample of fluid from the affected joints
- Blood culture

Osteoarthritis

- X-ray shows loss of joint space and formation of marginal osteophyte

Consult a Doctor if

- Pain and stiffness come on quickly, whether from an injury or an unknown cause
- A child has swinging fever, weight loss and loss of appetite associated with pain or a rash on armpits, knees, wrists, and ankles
- Joint pain associated with fever
- Pain and stiffness in the morning

Treatment and Management

In all cases of arthritis, generally, we use three stage therapy which consists of *medication* to relieve pain and inflammation, *rest* to let the injured tissues heal themselves, and *exercise* to rebuild strength and mobility.

Homoeopathy

+ For external application use Rhus tox. ointment or Ruta ointment and mother tincture of Stellaria media

There are many remedies for all type of arthritic pain. Following an analysis of overall situation, you can take remedies that may relieve pain and other symptoms. The following remedies are commonly used in arthritis:

Bryonia Alba 30

4 pills three times daily for one month

Symptoms

+ *Joint red, hot, swollen with stitches and tearing*
+ Knees stiff and painful
+ Every spot is painful on pressure
+ During sprain and strain, joint is painful and swollen, distended with fluid with great stiffness
+ Weariness and heaviness in all limbs and stiffness
+ Swelling of elbow extending as far as the middle of upper arm and of forearm
+ Swollen sensation in joints of finger on writing or taking hold of anything with pain
+ Heaviness and weakness of legs while walking and on standing

Arthritis

- Stitching pain in hip joint extending to knees
- Weariness of thigh worse with ascending stairs, better descending
- *Constant motion of left arm and leg*

The following symptoms generally accompany the above symptoms . . .

- Dryness of all mucous membranes like lips, mouth, throat, nose, chest, digestive tract
- *Excessive thirst.* Drinks large quantity of cold water
- Symptoms develop slowly
- Patient is irritable
- Patient wants to be left alone, wants to go home even when at home
- Delirium—talks of business
- Complaints which come on *after humiliation and anger*
- Right-sided complaints
- Physical weakness
- Nausea and faintness when rising up
- Pressure in stomach after eating, as of a stone
- Bursting, splitting headache

Symptoms *Worse*

- From least motion and touch, by change of position, by any effort to talk, to cough, even by moving eye balls and by winking
- Hot weather after a cold spell and warmth
- Intolerance of heat
- After eating
- Exertion
- Suppressed perspiration

Symptoms *Better*

- Hard pressure and rest
- Lying on the painful side
- From perspiring
- Cold things, cold air, cold water
- Darkened room

- Breast hot and painful, hard
- Chest painful while coughing
- Constipation, *stool hard, dry, dark, as if burnt*
- *Stitches* and stiffness in small of back
- Cough, dry, spasmodic with gagging and vomiting, after eating and drinking

Rhus Toxicodendron 30

4 pills three times daily for one month

Symptoms

- Hot, painful swelling of joint
- Tearing and drawing pain
- *Limbs stiff, paralysed sensation*
- Tenderness about knee joint
- Trembling after exertion
- Tingling in feet
- Loss of power in forearm and fingers
- Crawling sensation in the tips of finger
- *Tearing pain in tendons, ligament and fasciae*
- Numbness after over work and exposure
- Soreness of condyles of bones
- Pains aching, sore, bruised, tearing, shooting with heaviness, lameness and stiffness

Symptoms *Worse*

- The cold, fresh air is not tolerable
- Damp weather and after rains
- From sitting and rising from sitting position or first attempt to move
- Approach of storms
- At night, especially in bed
- After overwork and exposure
- From gardening
- Checked perspiration
- Injuries after lifting and over exertion

Arthritis

- *Sprains, strains, torn ligaments and tendinitis*

The following symptoms generally accompany the above symptoms...

- *Extreme restlessness* accompanies most symptoms. Cannot stay in one position, continued changes of position
- Aching in bone with fever
- Tongue coated, except red triangular space at tip with great thirst
- Bitter taste in mouth
- Skin eruptions—red, swollen with intense itching
- Desire for milk
- Fever of typhoid character
- General or localised glandular swelling
- Trembling and palpitation of heart when siting still
- *Sensitive to open air,* putting the hand from under the bedcover brings on cough

Symptoms *Better*
• From external heat
• Warm compresses
• From warmth of bed
• Continued movement
• Change of position
• Moving affected part
• Rubbing
• From stretching out limbs

Ledum Palustre 30

4 pills three times daily for one month

Symptoms

- It is a very good remedy for *rheumatic* and *arthritic* infections in both acute and chronic form

Symptoms *Worse*
• At night
• From warmth of bed and bed covering
• From motion
• While walking
• From alcohol
• Towards evening

- All the joints (like hips, knees, shoulders) are affected but especially small joints
- *Rheumatism begins in feet and travels upwards* and may even affect the heart
- Tearing, shooting, stinging and oppressive type of pain
- Throbbing in right shoulder
- Pressure in shoulder on raising or moving the arm
- Joint swollen, hot and pale without fever
- Cracking in joints
- Pain in right hip
- Stiffness of knee with weakness and trembling when walking
- Trembling of hands on moving them or grasping anything
- *Soles painful*, can hardly step on them
- Ankles swollen
- *Gouty pains* shoot all through the foot and limbs and in joints
- Ball of great toe swollen
- Gout begins in lower limb and ascends
- Gouty deposits in wrists, fingers and toes
- Easy s*praining* of ankle
- Injured part feels cold or numb yet pains are better from cold application

Symptoms *Better*
• Cold application
• Putting feet in cold water
• From getting out of bed
• Rest
• In cool air
• From copious urination with red or pale deposits

Arthritis

The following symptoms generally accompany the above symptoms...

- There is a *general lack of animal heat,* feels chilly all the time
- Patient is irritable, desires to be alone
- The *parts affected are cold* to touch but not felt cold by the patient. He feels *better by cold application*
- Wounded parts are cold. Punctured wounds from nails or splinter and insect stings
- *Red pimples on forehead and cheeks*
- Anal fissures
- Severe bruises or black eye with discoloration of the area. Bruises that feel cold and numb.

Colchicum 30

4 pills three times daily for one month

Symptoms

- Very good remedy for *gout*
- Inflammation of big toe and heel
- Acute pain making patient scream when touched
- Tearing, stitching, jerking pains especially in finger joints
- Pains go from left to right
- Skin rose coloured, leaves a white spot under the pressure of the finger
- Metastasis from big toe to heart
- Shifting *rheumatism* present, generally small joint affected. *Pain shifting from one joint to another*
- Joint stiff and fever is, tender and swollen
- Pains are shooting, tearing and twitches like electric shock

- Rheumatic pains all over the body—arms, back, neck and shoulder
- Swelling of the affected joint is red or pale with extreme tenderness
- Sensation of pin and needles in hands and wrist, fingertips numb
- Tingling in finger nails
- Knee strike together, can hardly walk
- Oedematous swelling pits on pressure
- Pain in front of thigh
- Sharp pain down left arm
- Limbs weak, lame and tingling
- Cramps of calves

The following symptoms generally accompany the above symptom...

- There is always great prostration, internal coldness and tendency to collapse
- Violence of all symptoms, worse between sundown to sunrise
- *The smell of fluid causes nausea even fainting;* he gags from mere mention of food especially fish, eggs

Symptoms *Worse*

- From least touch and slightest motion, cannot bear to have it touched or moved
- Sundown to sunrise
- Motion
- Loss of sleep
- In autumn
- In evening
- Smell of food under preparation or strong odours
- Mental exertion
- Suppressed perspiration
- Cold, wet weather

Symptoms *Better*

- Sitting
- Rest
- Stooping
- Rubbing
- Warmth
- From doubling up

Arthritis

- ✦ Great icy coldness in stomach
- ✦ Unquenchable thirst for cold drinks, alcoholic beverages
- ✦ Distension of abdomen, with gas, inability to stretch out legs
- ✦ Autumnal dysentery, stool shreddy and bloody

Causticum 30

4 pills three times daily for one month

Symptoms

- ✦ It is mainly useful in chronic rheumatic, arthritic and paralytic affections
- ✦ Generally indicated by tearing, drawing pains in the muscular and fibrous tissues, with deformities about the joints, especially knee and shoulder joint
- ✦ Restlessness in night with tearing pain of joints
- ✦ Pains are severe, generally remain in one joint for a long time
- ✦ Joints are stiff
- ✦ *Rheumatic tearing in limbs*
- ✦ Burning in joints
- ✦ Dull and tearing pain in hands and arm
- ✦ Rheumatism of the jaw with great stiffness

Symptoms *Worse*
- In dry, cold wind
- In clear, fine weather
- Cold air
- From motion of carriage
- Expectoration
- Walking
- New moon
- After stools

Symptoms *Better*
- By warmth, especially heat of bed
- In damp, wet weather
- Open air
- Stooping low
- Emission of flatus

- Unsteadiness of *muscles of forearm* and hands
- Numbness, loss of sensation in hands
- Rheumatic pain of shoulders, cannot raise hand, painful stiffness between scapulae
- Pain in nape of neck as from bruises
- *Contracted tendons*
- Weak ankles, cannot walk without suffering
- Unsteady walking and easy falling
- *Restless legs at night.* Cannot find a position to lie still in bed for a moment at night
- Cracking and tension in knees, stiffness in hollow of knee
- Painful stiffness in the limbs through the hips, especially on rising from a seat or from a recumbent position
- Itching on the dorsum of feet

The following symptoms generally accompany the above symptoms . . .

- Causticum patient is sad, hopeless, dark complexioned and *intensely sympathetic*
- *Burning, rawness* and *soreness* are characteristic
- General tendency of paralytic affection
- Restlessness at night and faint-like sinking of strength. Thus weakness progresses towards paralysis
- Paralysis of single parts—vocal cards, muscles of swallowing, of tongue, eyelids, face, bladder and extremities
- Dirty white sallow skin with warts especially on the face
- Symptoms worse on right side of body
- *Coryza with hoarseness*
- *Pimples and warts* on nose

- ✦ Aversion to sweets
- ✦ Thirst for cold water but aversion to drinking
- ✦ Menses cease at night, *flow only during day*
- ✦ *Hoarseness* with pain in chest and *loss of voice*
- ✦ Cough with *raw soreness of chest*
- ✦ Expectoration scanty, must be swallowed
- ✦ Cough with *pain in hip*, worse in evening, *better with drinking cold water*
- ✦ Difficulty of voice of singers and public speakers
- ✦ *Warts* large, bleeding easily, on tips of fingers and nose
- ✦ *Retention of urine*
- ✦ Bed wetting soon after falling asleep (during first sleep)
- ✦ Involuntary urine may also dribble while coughing or sneezing or after any excitement
- ✦ Constant mental stress, effects of shock or grief, any long standing worry

Magnesia Phosphorica 30

4 tablets three times daily for one month

Symptoms
- ✦ Neuralgic pain and cramping of muscles
- ✦ In sprain and strain sharp, stabbing, shooting pain
- ✦ Pain generally sharp, cutting, piercing, knife like, stabbing, shooting, stitching, lightening like
- ✦ Involuntary shaking of hands

Symptoms *Worse*
• On the right side
• Touch
• Night
• Cold bathing or washing
• Being uncovered
• Walking in fresh air

- Cramps in calves
- Writer's and player's cramp
- Weakness in arms and legs
- Finger tips numb and stiff
- General muscular weakness

Symptoms *Better*
• Warmth and heat
• Bending double
• Pressure
• Friction

The following symptoms generally accompany the above symptoms . . .

- Suitable for lean thin emaciated persons who are forgetful, easily tired, drowsy, averse to mental effort
- Main remedy for *spasmodic pain; pain generally sudden and severe*
- Painful ailment relieved by the *application of heat*
- Pain shifts rapidly and usually affects right side of the body
- Craving for sugar, averse to coffee
- May have thirst for cold drinks
- *Menstrual cramping* better after the flow begins
- Indicated for *all forms of cramp,* spasmodic and neuralgic pains in head, face, teeth, abdomen or stomach
- A fine remedy for the tummy pains of babies
- Flatulent colic, forcing the patient to bend double, accompanied with belching of gas, which gives no relief. Bloated abdomen, must loosen cloth, walk about and constantly pass flatus
- Spasmodic cough, whooping cough
- Angia pectoris
- In fever, chills run up and down the back with shivering
- Great dread of cold air, *of uncovering,* of touching the affected part, of cold bathing or walking, moving

Pulsatilla 30

4 pills three times daily for one month

Symptoms

- ✦ Drawing, tearing pains in joints with swelling and *redness*, especially hips, knees, elbows and small joints of hand and feet
- ✦ The *pains shift* rapidly *from one part to another*
- ✦ Can hardly give symptoms and starts crying
- ✦ Rheumatic pains are so severe that the patient is compelled to move slowly, as easy motion relieves
- ✦ Drawing, tensive pain in thighs and legs with restlessness and *chilliness*
- ✦ *Pain in limbs*, tensive pain, *letting up with a snap*
- ✦ Pain appears in a part, increases to a climax and then disappears suddenly from the part
- ✦ Pain in limbs in the morning in bed on walking with stiffness
- ✦ Hip-joint painful
- ✦ Knees swollen, with tearing, drawing pains
- ✦ Boring pain in heels like pricking of nails towards evening, *suffering worse from letting the affected limb hang down*
- ✦ Feet red inflamed and swollen

Symptoms *Worse*

- From heat
- Rich fat food
- After eating
- In warm close room
- Evening
- At twilight
- Lying on left or on the painless side
- When allowing feet to hang down
- At beginning to move
- On being seated or flexing (back)

- Numbness around elbow
- Tearing in the shoulder joint obliging him to bend arms, extends intermittently to wrists and fingers
- Legs feel heavy and weary
- Nervousness, intensely felt about the ankles

The following symptoms generally accompany the above symptoms . . .

- Very often indicated in the later, established stage of illness
- It is pre-eminently a female remedy, especially for mild, gentle, sad, crying, readily *weeps when talking, changeable,* contradictory
- Feels better by consolation
- The patient is chilly but she *feels better in open air and seeks the open air*
- Dry mouth but absence of thirst with nearly all complaints
- *Secretion* from all mucous membranes are *thick, bland and yellowish-green*
- *Symptoms ever changing*—no two stools, no two attacks alike; very well one hour, very miserable the next
- Pains *rapidly shifting* from one part to another
- Eyes inflamed and agglutinated, styes
- Cracks in middle of lower lips. *Yellow or white tongue*, covered with a tenacious mucous
- Desire for rich and fatty food, which leads to indigestion

Symptoms *Better*

- Cool open air
- Slow motion
- Cold application
- Cold food and drink
- Lying on the painful side
- Pressure or tying up tightly especially in head
- Rest

Arthritis

- Dry cough in the evening and at night, must sit up in bed to get relief and loose cough in the morning. Pressure upon the chest and soreness
- Menses too late, scanty or suppressed
- Useful remedy to begin the treatment in a chronic case

Aconite Napellus 30

4 pills three times daily for one month

Symptoms

- It is useful in sudden onset of an *acute rheumatism* and *acute arthritis*
- Sudden onset of disease with fever
- *Numbness and tingling*, shooting pains, icy coldness and insensibility of hands and feet
- Bruised feeling over entire body
- Heaviness of all limbs
- Arms feel lame bruised, heavy, numb
- Pain down the left arm
- *Hot hands* and *cold feet*
- Swelling of hands
- Numbness and tingling in fingers
- Rheumatic inflammation of joints, red shining swelling, very sensitive to contact
- Weak and lax ligaments of all joints

Symptoms *Worse*

- In evening and night about midnight
- In warm room
- Lying on the affected side
- From severe cold weather and dry cold winds
- From music
- From intense heat especially sun's heat
- Hot days and cold night
- Warm covering
- From tobacco-smoke

- ✦ Painless cracking of all joints
- ✦ Hip joint and thigh feels lame, especially after lying down
- ✦ Knees unsteady, disposition of foot to turn
- ✦ Sensation as if drops of water have trickled down the thigh
- ✦ Rheumatism with fever; fever high grade with restlessness, fear and anxiety of mind and nervous excitability. The patient is unappeasable, tossing about with agony, skin hot and dry but sweat drenching on parts laid on

Symptoms *Better*
• Open air
• Rest
• By uncovering
• Sitting still
• After perspiration

The following symptoms generally accompany the above symptoms . . .

- ✦ *Physical and mental restlessness* is the most characteristic symptom of Aconite
- ✦ *Acute and sudden onset and violent invasion with fever*
- ✦ *Complaints and tension* caused by exposure to dry *cold weather*, draught of cold air, checked perspiration and also from very *hot weather*
- ✦ Great *fear, anxiety* and worry accompany every ailment
- ✦ *Fear of death, fear the future*
- ✦ Its action is brief and *shows no marked periodicity*
- ✦ Burning thirst—for large quantity
- ✦ *Heavy,* pulsating, *hot, bursting* headache
- ✦ Vertigo, *worse on rising*
- ✦ Very sensitive to light, music, smell, touch and pain
- ✦ Burning in internal parts, *tingling, numbness and coldness*

Arthritis

- Tongue coated white
- Vomiting, with fever, heat, profuse sweat and increased urination
- Urine scanty, red, hot and painful
- *Oppressed breathing* on least motion. *Hoarse, dry, croupy cough*
- Shortness of breath, cough worse *at night* and *after midnight*
- *Palpitation with anxiety* and tingling in finger
- Fever with *great thirst* for cold water and *restlessness*. Cold waves pass through him
- Most complaints disappear when sitting still

Arnica Montana 30

4 pills three times daily for one month

Symptoms

- Rheumatism of muscular and tendinous tissue, especially of hip, back and shoulders
- It is suited to cases when any injury, however remote, seems to have caused the present trouble *After traumatic injury*
- A muscular tonic
- Limbs and body aches as if beaten joints, as if sprained
- *Sore, lame and brushed feeling*
- Sharp, shooting, paralytic or sprained pains which quickly change place

Symptoms *Worse*
• With least touch
• Motion
• Rest
• Wine
• Damp cold
• Evening
• From speaking
• Blowing nose
• Almost any noise
• Lying on injured part
• From over-exertion
• Alcohol
• Old age

- *Gouty affections.* Great fear at being touched or approached
- Sore, tender, red swelling of the joints in gout particularly of knee joint
- Gout with arthritic pains in the feet and the big toe as if sprained
- In arthritis especially hip joint is affected
- Rheumatism begins low down and works up
- Cannot walk erect, on account of bruised pain in pelvic region
- Paralytic pains in all joints during motion
- Knee bends suddenly when walking, stitches when touched
- Twitching pain from left shoulder, joint to middle finger
- Pain in back and limbs, as if bruised
- Deathly coldness of forearms
- Everything on which he lies seems too hard
- Soreness after over-exertion
- Cracking in the right wrist when the hand is moved, as if dislocated
- During *Sprains* and *Strains* ligaments torn with swelling which is most prominent. Bruising and inflammation of the soft tissue around the joint
- When muscles or soft tissues are black and blue

Symptoms *Better*
• Lying down
• Lying with head low
• Warmth
• Rubbing and wrapping up warmly
• Long walk in cold weather
• Out stretched
• By changing position

Following symptoms generally accompany the above symptoms . . .
- Produces conditions similar to those resulting from injuries, falls, blows, contusions
- Especially suited to cases when any injury occurs. *After any traumatic injuries*
- Remote effects of injuries even though received years ago
- Whole body feels *sore and bruised, lame* and does not want to be approached, touched or jarred
- It *promotes healing,* reduces swelling, prevents pus formation
- It is very effective in bleeding of any kind
- *Head hot with cold body*
- Fetid breath
- Diarrhoea offensive and bloody
- *Violent spasmodic cough with facial herpes*
- Skin *black and blue*. Multiple small boils very painful. Acne characterised by *symmetry in distribution*
- *Aids recovery after an operation*

Calcarea Phosphorica 30
4 pills three times daily for one month

Symptoms
- Shooting, tearing and aching type of rheumatic pain in all parts of body especially knees, loins and thumb
- Pain with stiffness, coldness, *numbness and crawling sensation*
- Pain become worse by any change of weather
- Buttocks, back and limbs fall asleep

- ✦ Weary when going upstairs. Cannot rise from seat. Staggering in old people when rising from a seat
- ✦ Pain in joints and bones excited or increased by every draft of cold damp air
- ✦ Rheumatism of cold weather, getting well in spring and symptoms return in autumn

The following symptoms generally accompany the above symptom . . .

- ✦ For anaemic persons, especially *anaemic children* who are flabby, have cold extremities and feeble digestion
- ✦ Children—*emaciated, unable to stand, and slow in learning to walk*
- ✦ *Feels complaints more when thinking about them*
- ✦ *Numbness and crawling* are characteristic sensations
- ✦ Symptoms get worse by wet cold air and every *change of weather*
- ✦ Headache, *worse near the region of sutures*
- ✦ Glandular enlargement—swollen tonsils. *Adenoid growths*
- ✦ *Craving for bacon, ham, salted or smoked meat*
- ✦ *Much flatulence.* Flatulence temporarily relieved by sour eructations

Symptoms *Worse*
- Exposure to cold and damp weather
- Cold air
- Melting snow
- Changeable weather
- East winds
- Mental exertion
- Dinner
- After a meal, especially juicy fruits
- Motion

Symptoms *Better*
- In summer
- Warm, dry atmosphere
- Lying down
- Rest
- Passing wind

Arthritis

- Pain in abdomen *at every attempt to eat*
- Diarrhoea from juicy fruits, during dentition *with fetid flatus*
- White discharge in females, *like white of egg*

Kali Iodide 30
4 pills three times daily for one month

Symptoms

- Rheumatic pain at night and in damp weather
- *Rheumatism of knee with effusion*
- Severe bone pains. Gnawing pain in left leg. Bones are sensitive to touch especially shin bone (leg bone)
- Contractions of joints
- Pain is hips causes limping when walking
- Gout affecting every joint with an indication that hepatic region is painful on touch
- Sensation as if small insects were crawling on the skin of lower extremities when sitting, better lying down
- Rheumatism in *neck, back,* feet especially heels and soles worse cold and wet

Symptoms *Worse*
- Warm clothing
- Warm room
- At night
- Damp, wet weather
- Touch
- At rest
- Lying on painful side or on back

Symptoms *Better*
- Open air (walking in open air dose not fatigue)
- Motion

The following symptoms generally accompany the above symptoms . . .

- It acts prominently on fibrous and connective tissues, producing infiltration oedema
- *Glandular swelling*
- Emaciation and weakness
- Headache at *sides* and *root of nose*
- Profuse, *acrid, hot, watery, thin* discharge from nose
- Saliva increased, cold food and drink, especially milk, increases the suffering
- *Larynx feel raw.* Awakes choking *Expectoration like soap-suds, greenish*
- Pimples with red tip

Guaiacum ϕ

10 drops (mix with water) two times daily for one month

Symptoms

- Its main action is on fibrous tissue, that is why it is adopted to arthritic and rheumatic complaints
- It is very valuable in *acute rheumatism*
- Rheumatic pain in shoulders, arms and hands
- Joints swollen, painful and intolerant of pressure, cannot bear heat
- Stinging pain in limbs

Symptoms *Worse*

- Heat
- From motion
- Cold wet weather
- Pressure
- Touch
- From 6 p.m. to 4 a.m.
- When sitting
- In the morning, immediately on rising
- In evening before going to sleep

- ✦ Arthritic lancination followed by contraction of limbs
- ✦ *A feeling* of *heat* in the affected limbs

Symptoms *Better*
- External pressure

- ✦ Gouty tearing with contraction. Immovable stiffness
- ✦ *Gouty and rheumatic pain in head* and face, *extending to neck*
- ✦ Ankle pain extending up the leg, causing lameness
- ✦ Contraction of limbs, stiffness and immobility. Feeling that one must stretch
- ✦ *Growing pains*
- ✦ Aching in bones
- ✦ *Stiff neck and sore shoulder*

Following symptoms generally accompany the above symptoms...

- ✦ It has *free foul secretions* and *unclean odour* from the whole body
- ✦ Promotes suppuration of abscess
- ✦ *Acute tonsillitis.* Throat dry and burn
- ✦ *Desire for apples* and other fruits. Aversion to milk
- ✦ Patient feels as if the eyes are swollen and protruded and the lids appear too short to cover them
- ✦ *Feels suffocated*

Rhododendron 30
4 pills three times daily for one month

Symptoms
- ✦ Well marked *rheumatic and gouty* symptoms
- ✦ It affects *mainly small joints*

- Joints are red and swollen
- *Rheumatic tearing* in *all limbs,* especially in the right side
- Numbness and formication
- Rheumatic pain in bones in spots and reappears with change of weather
- Pain in shoulders, arms and wrists
- Pain in limbs especially felt in the forearm and leg down to the fingers and toes
- Digging, drawing, sprained pains in wrists
- Heaviness, weakness and tremors in hand
- Paralytic pain in right shoulder when resting open it, sometimes extending below elbow
- Heaviness in thighs. Pain in hips as if sprained
- *Cannot sleep unless legs are crossed*
- Gouty inflammation of great toe-joint with swelling and redness
- Acute and chronic gouty conditions

Symptoms *Worse*
• Before a storm
• All symptoms reappear in rough weather
• Windy weather
• Wet cold weather
• Night
• Towards morning
• Rest
• Wine

Symptoms *Better*
• After a storm breaks
• Warmth
• Dry heat
• Exercise
• By eating
• From wrapping the head
• Immediately on starting to move

The following symptoms generally accompany the above symptoms...

- Patient is gloomy, forgetful and afraid of thunderstorm

- All symptoms worse before a storm, relieved when it breaks
- Pain in lower jaw and chin, better with *warmth* and *eating*
- Testicles intensely painful to touch, drawn up, swollen and painful. Hydrocoele

Kalmia Latifolia 30
4 pills three times daily for one month

Symptoms

- It is a rheumatic remedy with *rapidly shifting pains*, going from joint to joint
- Joints red, hot, swollen and pain worse form least movement
- If rheumatism is suppressed by external application to the affected part, then there is metastasis to the heart
- Pains and aching in limbs accompanying every symptom
- Pain travels downward from above
- Tearing pain with numbness, tingling, trembling and weakness, especially left arm
- Pain from hips to knee and feet
- Pain *affects a large part of a limb*, or several joints, and pass through quickly
- Weakness, numbness, pricking and sense of coldness in limbs

Symptoms *Worse*
- Leaning forward
- Looking down
- Open air
- Motion
- Exertion

Symptoms *Better*
- Eating food
- Continued motion
- Profuse urination (especially headache)

- Pain in left shoulder with pressure in left arm, in left elbow extending to the wrist or to the little finger
- Pain *along ulnar nerve*, index finger
- Gout, affecting fingers mostly
- Rheumatic chest pains
- The rheumatic pains are mostly in the upper part of the arms and lower parts of the legs and are worse when going to sleep

The following symptoms generally accompany the above symptoms . . .

- Rheumatic pain maybe accompanied by nausea and slow pulse
- It has a prominent action on the heart
- Neuralgia, *pains shoot downward with numbness*
- Facial neuralgia especially on right side
- Vertigo, *movement of eyes painful*
- Pain in pit of stomach, worse with bending forewards, relieved by sitting erect
- Weak, slow pulse
- Palpitation, *worse leaning foreward*
- Sharp pain, in heart region, take away the breath
- Shooting through chest above the heart into shoulder-blades
- Sleepless, wakes very early in morning

Chelidonium Majus 30

4 pills three times daily for one month

Symptoms

- A prominent liver remedy, that's why rheumatic and arthritic complaints generally associated with hepatic derangement

Arthritis

- ✦ It covers acute cases of rheumatism with oedema, heat, tenderness and stiffness especially feet and ankles. The pains get worse by the least touch and slightest movement, generally patients screams with pain
- ✦ Rheumatic pain in hips and thighs
- ✦ Shooting pain in the right hip, may radiate into the abdomen
- ✦ Intolerable pains in heels, as if pinched by too narrow a shoe, worse on right side better by bathing with warm water
- ✦ Wandering cramp-like pains in all over body, in limbs, shoulder, arms, hands, tips of fingers with soreness on contact
- ✦ *Icy coldness of tips of fingers*
- ✦ Wrist painful, tearing in bones of hand
- ✦ Pain all over in joints and bones as if sprained, better from pressure
- ✦ Tearing pain and stiffness in small of back
- ✦ *Fixed pain under inner and lower angle of right scapula*
- ✦ Rigidity of muscles in lower limbs

Symptoms *Worse*
• On the right side
• Slightest motion
• Least touch
• Very early morning
• In the afternoon
• Change of weather

Symptoms *Better*
• From pressure
• After dinner
• After rest
• Bathing the affected part constantly with hot water

The following symptoms generally accompany the above symptoms . . .

- ✦ A prominent liver remedy, especially constant pain under inferiors angle of right scapula

- Affects right side most: right eye, right lung, right side of abdomen, right hip and leg
- Complaints brought on or renewed by change of weather, and after dinner
- Face yellow
- Desire of hot food and drinks
- Eating relieves temporarily, especially when complaint is accompanied with hepatic symptoms
- Alternation of diarrhoea and constipation
- Yellow-gray colour of skin

Formica Ruta 30

4 pills three times daily for one month

Symptoms

- Mainly an arthritic remedy
- Right side most commonly affected
- Chronic gout and stiffness in joints
- Some time acute attack of gout pain; pain worse with motion; pain better with pressure
- Rheumatic pain—stiff and contracted joints
- *Rheumatic complaints come suddenly with restlessness; sweat does not relieve any complaints*

Symptoms Worse
• Cold and cold washing
• Dampness
• Before a snow-storm
• On the right side
• Motion
• Sitting

Symptoms Better
• Warmth
• Pressure
• Rubbing
• After midnight
• Combing hair

Arthritis

- Muscles feel strained and torn from their attachment
- Complaints from over lifting
- *Weakness of lower extremities*
- Pain in hips
- Paralysis of all limbs

The following symptoms generally accompany the above symptoms . . .

- Cracking in left ear with headache
- Coryza and stopped-up feeling in nose
- It has marked deterrent influence on the formation of polypi
- Pain in bowels before stool
- Drawing pain around navel before stool
- Skin—red, itching and burning
- Nodes around joints
- Profuse sweat without relief

Lycopodium 30
4 pills three times daily for one month

Symptoms

- It is useful in chronic rheumatism and arthritis
- Rheumatic pain may occur in any of the joints of the body but knee and finger joints are commonly affected
- Numbness, drawing and tearing in limbs especially while at rest or at night
- Pain will often have started on right-side of body and moved over to the left
- Spasmodic contraction and extension without pain
- Pains come and go suddenly

- ✦ Heaviness of arms
- ✦ Tearing pain in shoulder and elbow joints
- ✦ Tearing pain in joints with stiffness
- ✦ *Chronic gout,* with chalky deposits in joints with urinary trouble; red sand and clear urine
- ✦ Gout which affects especially the right side
- ✦ Pain in heel on treading as from a pebble
- ✦ Profuse sweat on the feet
- ✦ Hands and feet numb
- ✦ Swelling of feet, worse on the right side
- ✦ Cramps in calves and toes at night in bed
- ✦ Twitching and jerking

Symptoms *Worse*
• From right to left
• From above leading downwards
• 4 to 8 p.m.
• At night
• From heat or warm room
• Hot air
• Warmth of bed
• Warm application (expect throat and stomach which are better from warm drinks)
• On beginning to move

The following symptoms generally accompany the above symptoms . . .

- ✦ In nearly all cases where Lycopodium is the remedy, some evidence of urinary or digestive disturbance will be found
- ✦ Ailment develops gradually
- ✦ A *right-sided* remedy, complaints travel from right to left or from above leading downwards
- ✦ Symptoms are generally *worse* from *4 p.m. to 8 p.m*
- ✦ Its patient is generally lean, flatulent, has wrinkles and *prematurely old*

Arthritis

- Carving for sweets and warm food and drinks
- Patient is *apprehensive, afraid to be alone,* spells or writes wrong words
- Although *hungry but eating ever so little (few bites) create fullness*
- Food tastes sour
- Blisters on tongue
- Abdomen is bloated, full due to accumulation of wind, coupled with rumbling, gurgling and distension
- Stool hard, difficult to expel
- Dark, scanty urine, red sand in urine, frequency of urination increased at night
- Impotency in males

Symptoms *Better*
• From continued motion
• After midnight
• Stomach and throat complaint relieved by warm drinks and food
• On getting cold
• In cool open air
• On being uncovered

Sulphur 30
4 pills twice daily for fifteen days

Symptoms
- Rheumatic and arthritic complaints due to suppression of any skin disease
- *Painful stiffness* is main symptom, with or without effusion
- For preventing gouty diathesis there is no better remedy than *Sulphur*
- One of the leading remedy for synovitis
- *Hot, sweaty hands*
- Trembling of hands

- Sprained pain in wrist
- Pain in left shoulder as if joint is dislocated
- Jerking in deltoid
- Drawing pain in shoulder and arms
- Swelling in fingers in morning, sticking in tips at night; of flexure surface of right middle finger
- *Stooping shoulders*, cannot walk erect
- Tearing above the nail of left ring finger, worse in the evening
- Sharp drawing, shooting and stitches here and there
- Pains seem to ascend, is worse in mid summer heat, on clear and cloudless days
- Sweat in armpits, smelling like garlic
- Stiffness of knees and ankles
- *Burning in soles and hands at night*
- Weakness of thighs and legs
- Tearing extending into middle of thigh, worse standing and on ascending stairs
- Tearing through knee extending to feet when walking and sitting
- Sprained wrenching pain in joints with cracking and stiffness, particularly in knees and shoulders

Symptoms *Worse*
- At rest
- Around 11 a.m.
- In the morning
- At night
- Warmth of bed
- When standing
- Washing and bathing
- From alcoholic stimulants
- From weather changes
- Periodically

Symptoms *Better*
- Dry, warm weather
- In open air
- Lying on right side
- From drawing up affected limbs

Arthritis

- Sudden cramp-like, painful jerking about the hip joints with stiffness
- Tension, pain in joints on walking
- Tension in hollow of knees, as if too short, on stepping
- Inclination to cramp on stretching out feet
- Rheumatic gout with itching
- Swelling and inflammation of big toe with pain

The following symptoms generally accompany the above symptoms...

- Burning everywhere in the body especially in the head, palm and sole
- *Dirty, filthy people,* prone to skin disease, dry and hard hair and skin
- Children—*cannot bear to be washed or bathed*
- Aversion of being washed
- *When carefully selected remedies fail to produce a favourable effect,* especially in acute disease
- Itching eruption on the skin. Scratching is followed by burning
- *Standing is worse position* for patients, they cannot stand
- *Complaints are relapsing*—the patient seems to get almost well but the disease returns
- Redness of all orifices (lips, ears, eyelids, nostrils, anus, urethra etc.) as if pressed full of blood
- Discharges are offensive in character
- The discharges both of urine and faeces is painful to parts over which it passes; *parts around anus red, excoriated.* All the orifices of the body are very red
- *Milk disagrees,* craves sugar, sweets and fatty food

- *Great acidity* and sour eructations
- *Diarrhoea,* painless, *driving out of bed early in the morning*
- *Weak, empty gone* feeling and *faint about 11 a.m.*

Arsenicum Album 30

4 pills three times daily for fifteen days

Symptoms

- Shin bones and knees are especially affected
- Trembling, twitching, spasms, weakness, heaviness and uneasiness present all over extremities
- Burning and tearing in limbs after previous over-exertion
- Cramps in calves
- Extreme restlessness in limbs, better by movement; sometimes he keeps his feet moving about while in bed
- Swelling of feet and legs
- Paralysis of lower limbs with atrophy
- Trembling and swollen hands
- Tearing in arms from elbow to shoulder
- Pain in the arm, on which he lies at night
- Pain in knee, as if beaten
- Swelling and pain in ankles

Symptoms *Worse*
• Cold and wet weather
• After midnight (particularly between midnight and 3 a.m.)
• From cold drinks or food
• Seashore
• After eating or drinking
• On the right side
• From lying with head low
• Physical exertion
• During sleep
• During stool
• After undressing
• Vomiting
• On awakening

Arthritis

- Sensation as if joints would break down when descending
- Ulcers on heel
- Sore pain in the ball of great toe, while walking

The following symptoms generally accompany the above symptoms...

- *Great exhaustion after the slightest exertion* and worse at night, with all complaints
- *Restlessness—mentally restless but physically too weak to move*
- *Burning pains*—the affected parts burn like fire, but relieved by heat, (except in head), hot drinks
- Patient is anxious, fearful and restless. *Changes place continually*
- Fear of death, thinks disease is incurable and he is going to die
- *Great thirst but drinks small quantity of water at short intervals*
- All symptoms are worse at midday and midnight (1 to 2 a.m./p.m.)
- Very fastidious patient, wants everything in order, neat and clean
- *Cannot bear the smell or sight of food*
- Periodicity, complaints returns annually
- Bad effects of vegetable diet, melons and watery fruits generally

Symptoms *Better*
• From heat
• From warm drinks
• On going down (descending)
• Lying with the head high
• Warm covers and warm application
• Changing position

- Stool *small, offensive, dark with much prostration,* worse at night and after eating and drinking
- Skin *dry, rough, scaly,* white spots on skin
- Fever—intermittent with marked exhaustion

Silica 30

4 pills three times daily for one month

Symptoms

- Mainly useful for the treatment of chronic rheumatism and arthritis
- Bruised pain in the whole body, in the morning before walking, better rising
- Bruised pain in all muscles of body
- Loss of power in legs
- Heaviness and weariness of lower limbs
- Pain in knee, as if tightly bound
- Calves tense and contracted
- Sole sores
- Soreness in feet
- Pain in great toes so that he can scarcely step on them
- Cramps in calves and soles
- *Icy cold and sweaty feet*
- Pain with weakness of joints, worse upper extremities or the ankle joint

Symptoms *Worse*
- In morning
- From washing
- From cold
- On uncovering
- Lying down
- Drafts of air
- At night
- Lying on the left side
- Mental work
- Motion
- New moon
- Change of weather
- Getting wet

Arthritis

- Biting pain in the hip extending to knee with tendency of bone pain and suppuration
- Tearing in the joint when sitting
- Cramp-like pain in the thumb joints
- Paralytic weakness of forearm
- Tremulous hands when using them
- Sensation in tips of fingers, as if suppurating.

Symptoms *Better*
• Warmth (all symptoms except gastric one which are better by cold food) • On wrapping up head • Summer

The following symptoms generally accompany the above symptoms . . .

- Useful in diseases of bones, caries and necrosis
- *Suppurative processes*, ripens abscesses since it promotes suppuration
- Ailment attended with *pus formation*
- Great sensitiveness of taking cold
- *Sensitive* to all impressions and *anxious*
- Headache better by *wrapping up warmly* and *when lying on the left side*
- Pain begins at back of the head, and spreads over head and settles over eyes
- *Profuse sweat of head*
- Tendency to inflammation, swelling and suppuration of glands—cervical, auxiliary, parotid, mammary. Small wounds heal with difficulty and suppurate easily
- *Pricking as if a pin in tonsil*

- ✦ Fissures and piles painful, with *spasm of sphincter of rectum*. Constipation, *stool* comes down *with difficulty, when partly expelled, recedes again*
- ✦ *Night walking*—gets up while asleep
- ✦ Violent *cough* when lying down with *thick, yellow lumpy* expectoration
- ✦ White spots on nails
- ✦ *Promotes expulsion of foreign bodies* from tissues, e.g. thorn, splinters.

Phytolacca 30

4 pills three times daily for one month

Symptoms

- ✦ It mainly acts well in chronic rheumatism
- ✦ A sore, bruised aching feeling all over the body; he feels he must move, movement increases his pain and soreness
- ✦ Rheumatic pain, worse in morning
- ✦ *Pains fly like electric shocks*
- ✦ Shooting, lancinating pain shifting rapidly
- ✦ Rheumatic swelling are hard, painful on touch and intensely hot
- ✦ Shooting pain in cardiac region alternating with pain in the right shoulder

Symptoms *Worse*
- In the morning on rising
- Sensitive to electric changes
- Effects of a wetting, when it rains
- Exposure to damp, cold weather
- Night
- Motion
- On the right side
- Hot drinks (especially in throat problem)

Arthritis

- Shooting pain in right shoulder, with stiffness and inability to raise arm
- Pain on undersides of thighs
- *Aching of heels,* relieved by elevating feet
- Pain in right knee in afternoon, worse in open air and damp weather
- Pain in legs, patient dreads to get up and move
- Pain like shocks
- Swelling in feet
- Pain in ankle and feet
- Neuralgic pain in big toes
- Rheumatism of fibrous and periosteal tissue

Symptoms *Better*
• Warmth
• Dry weather
• Rest

The following symptoms generally accompany the above symptoms . . .

- Aching, soreness, restlessness, weakness are guiding general symptoms
- Glandular swelling with heat and inflammation
- *Pain flying like electric shocks;* rapidly shifting pains
- *Increased secretion of tears*
- Right-sided remedy especially in throat
- *Children bite teeth or gums together* during teething
- *Throat feels rough, narrow,* hot. *Tonsils swollen*
- *Shooting pain into the ears on swallowing.* Cannot swallow anything hot
- Throat feels very hot, pain at roof of tongue extending to ear
- Urine scanty and suppressed with pain in kidney region

- ✦ *Breast hard, swollen and very sensitive*
- ✦ Disposition to boils

Stellaria Media 30

4 pills three times daily for one month; it can also be used as an external application (mother tincture) over the affected area.

Symptoms *Worse*
• With rest
• In the morning
• Warmth
• Tobacco

Symptoms *Better*
• In the evening
• Cold air
• Motion

Symptoms

- ✦ Sharp, *shifting rheumatic pains* all over the body
- ✦ Generally acts well in *chronic rheumatism*
- ✦ Sharp pain in small of the back, over kidney region, in gluteal region extending down the thigh
- ✦ *Rheumatism*—Darting pain all over the body with stiffness of joints
- ✦ Joint sore on touch, worse with motion
- ✦ Pain in shoulders and arms
- ✦ Rheumatic pain in calves
- ✦ Bruised feeling all over body
- ✦ *Synovitis*
- ✦ Gout—enlarged and inflamed finger joints

The following symptoms generally accompany the above symptoms . . .

- ✦ It includes a condition of stasis, congestion, and sluggishness of all function
- ✦ Mainly rheumatic and gout remedy

Arthritis

- General irritability. Indisposition to work
- Eyes feel protruded
- Neck muscles stiff and sore
- *Liver enlarged, swollen; stitching pain and sensitive to pressure*

Mercurius Solubilis 30
4 pills two times daily for one month

Symptoms

- It is more effective in case of acute gout
- Joints sore, pale, swollen and occasional tearing pain
- Fingers flexed especially thumb with difficulty in opening
- Weakness of limbs, he can scarcely walk
- Lancinating pain in joints
- Drawing rheumatic pain in long bones particularly where the skin is thin, worse at night
- *Trembling in extremities, especially hands,* and jerking of arms
- Boring pain in periosteum of right tibia (leg bone) and drawing pain in tibia
- Swelling of feet and leg
- Cold, clammy sweat on legs at night
- Tearing pain in hips and knees, worse in open air

Symptoms *Worse*
- At night
- Warmth of bed
- Warm room
- From lying on right side
- Wet, damp weather
- Extreme temperature
- Cold air, draft of air
- Sweating
- Daylight or firelight
- Before stool
- Sitting or walking
- During exercise

+ Painful stiffness of wrist
+ Rheumatic pain behind sternum, *cannot lie on the right side*

Symptoms *Better*
• In moderate temperature
• From rest
• During the day

The following symptoms generally accompany the above symptoms . . .

+ Complaints worse at night, from change of weather, and warmth of bed. He is *sensitive to extremes of cold and heat*
+ Glandular swelling with or without suppuration
+ Profuse and offensive sweating with complaints, complaints worse with the sweat
+ Intense thirst for cold water, with moist mouth with excessive saliva, which he is constantly swallowing
+ Discharges from all body increases and offensive
+ Fetid odour from mouth, metallic taste
+ Body smells offensive
+ Thick, moist coated tongue with imprint of teeth
+ *Tremors* and trembling everywhere from least exertion
+ Tension headache, *as if bandaged*
+ Gums spongy and bleed easily with pain on chewing
+ Dysentery *bloody, mucous stool* (more mucous than blood in stools), *with pain and tremors*
+ Skin almost constantly moist with marked tendency for ulcers, boils and pus formation in general
+ Emaciation with swelling of hands and feet, with anaemia

Actea Spicata 30

4 pills three times daily for one month

Symptoms

- Rheumatic remedy, especially affects *small joints, wrist,* fingers, *ankles*, toes
- Tearing, tingling pain
- Swelling of joints from slight fatigue
- *Wrist-rheumatism, wrist swollen,* red; worse during any motion
- Tearing pain in loins
- Pain in knees
- Lame feeling in arms
- Paralytic weakness in the hands
- Swelling of joint after little work

Symptoms *Worse*
• From touch
• Motion
• At night

The following symptoms generally accompany the above symptoms . . .

- Mainly rheumatic remedy
- Pulsation all over body, especially liver and renal region
- Vertigo, tearing headache
- Tearing, darting pains in epigastric region with vomiting
- Spasmodic retraction of abdomen
- *Great oppression. Shortness of breath on exposure to cold air*
- Short regular breathing at night, while lying

Belladonna 30

4 pills three times daily for one month

Symptoms

- It is a good remedy in acute and chronic rheumatism of an inflammatory nature
- Joints swollen, red and shining
- Shooting, tearing, aching, throbbing or bruise-like pain
- *Pain comes suddenly and disappears suddenly*
- Symptoms prefer the right side
- Shifting rheumatic pains means pain changes position from one joint to another
- Patient is extremely sensitive to touch or jar
- Shooting pain along limbs
- Jerking limbs
- Involuntary limping
- Pain with redness of eyes and face
- *Cold extremities*
- Oppressive, tearing pain in shoulders
- Paralytic twitching of arms with red swelling of hands and arms
- Paralytic feeling and weakness of whole left arm

Symptoms *Worse*

- In the afternoon, after 3 p.m.
- At night, especially after midnight
- Touching the affected part
- Jar
- Noise
- Draught of air
- Lying down
- Cold
- Uncovering head
- Sudden changes from warm to cold weather
- In hot weather
- Hot sun
- While looking at bright, shining object
- While drinking

Arthritis

- Tearing in middle joint of right index finger or in proximal joint of left middle finger
- Unsteady while walking
- Cutting stitches in outer muscles of right thigh, just above the knee, only when sitting
- Pain in thighs and legs as if caries
- When rising from bed, legs unable to carry the body weight and he sinks to the ground
- Stitches in hip joint, as if beaten

Symptoms *Better*
• Walking in open air
• When standing up after sitting
• While leaning the head against something
• Sitting erect
• Warm application (except in headache)
• Wrapping up
• In a warm room

The following symptoms generally accompany the above symptoms . . .

- Sudden and violent onset of disease which also disappears suddenly. *Pains come on suddenly and disappear suddenly*
- For inflammatory condition with heat, redness, throbbing and burning
- Complaints from cold, dry wind, especially from exposure of head to cold wind or getting head wet
- *Great children remedy*
- Redness of toes, eyes and of inflamed part
- Oversensitive to pain worse from slight touch, (worse from pressure of cloth, bed covering) slight movement and least jar
- Right sided remedy—Symptoms occur largely on the right side
- Great thirst for cold water but *anxiety or fear of drinking*

- ✦ Throat feels constricted, difficult in deglutition. Tonsils enlarged
- ✦ Retention of urine, *frequent and profuse urination*
- ✦ Menses too early, too profuse and very offensive and hot
- ✦ Ticking, short, dry cough, worse at night
- ✦ Glands *swollen, tender,* red. *Boils*
- ✦ Alternate redness and paleness of skin

Cinchona Officinalis 30
4 pills three times daily for one month

Symptoms
- ✦ It is more useful in chronic cases of gout and rheumatism
- ✦ *Pain in limbs and joints,* as if sprained, *worse with slight touch* and better by hard pressure
- ✦ Joint swollen and very sensitive with dread of open air
- ✦ Drawing and tearing pain in every joint
- ✦ Tendency of limbs to go to sleep
- ✦ Weakness of joints worse in the morning and when sitting
- ✦ Paralytic jerking and tearing in long bones, worse with touch
- ✦ Pain in thigh bone as if periosteum had been scraped with a dull knife

Symptoms *Worse*
- Slightest touch
- After eating
- At night
- Drafts of air
- Every other day
- Prolonged exertion
- Motion
- Loss of vital fluids
- Bending over
- From walking which makes the person dizzy
- From fruits and milk
- From perspiration

- Sensation as if string around limb
- Great debility, trembling and numb sensation
- Knees give away while walking, worse while ascending stairs
- Hot swelling of right knee with pain extending to thigh and leg
- Aversion to exercise and sensitive to touch
- Chronic synovitis of the knee
- In case of chronic gout when it is in monoarticular form and also during intervals between attacks
- One hand icy cold and other hand warm

Symptoms *Better*
• Bending double
• Hard pressure
• Warmth
• Open air
• Loose clothing
• Lying down

The following symptoms generally accompany the above symptoms . . .

- Ailments *from loss of vital fluids, especially haemorrhages,* excessive lactation, diarrhoea
- Symptoms with *marked periodicity,* return every other day, or regularly in season at same time
- Rapid general weakness with tendency of sweating from least excretion as well as sleep
- Patient is disobedient, depressed and ready to offend others
- Excessive *sensitivity to light, touch* but relief from hard pressure on painful part
- Throbbing headache, as if the skull would burst
- Excessive flatulence of stomach and bowels, belching gives no relief. Abdomen swollen like a drum with gas
- Frothy, watery, undigested stool; *painless diarrhoea*
- Passive haemorrhage from all outlets of the body with dark clotted blood

- *Intermittent fever worse every other day,* no thirst during heat, great thirst during sweat
- Anaemia and loss of appetite

Acid Benzoicum 30

4 pills three times daily for one month

Symptoms

- Useful in persons with *uric acid diathesis*
- It is a useful remedy in *gouty cases;* use it when Colchicum fails
- Swelling of the wrist with gout deposits
- Gouty deposits, nodes are very painful. Nodes on joints of fingers and toes
- Tearing pain in great toe
- *Bunion* of great toe
- Joint cracks on motion
- Tearing pain in tendons and joints with stitches
- *Pain in tendo-achilles*
- Pain and swelling in knees
- Oedema of the lower extremities
- Pain changes position suddenly, metastasise with heart pain in the cardiac region
- Rheumatism and gout alternate with heart trouble with pain in cardiac region

Symptoms *Worse*
• In open air
• By uncovering
• Cold air
• Change in weather
• Motion
• Wine
• Urine scanty

Symptoms *Better*
• By heat
• Profuse urination

The following symptoms generally accompany the above symptoms . . .

- *Offensive* odour of urine accompanies all symptoms
- Urine is scanty, of a dark brown colour with repulsive odour, the smell exists at the time of urination and stays long afterwards
- Dribbling of urine in old men with enlarged prostate
- Renal insufficiency. Renal colic
- Rheumatism and gout alternate with heart trouble with palpitation and pain in the cardiac region
- Stool offensive and liquid

Caulophyllum 30

4 pills three times daily for one month or Caulophyllum mother tincture, 15 drops in luke warm water two times daily for one month.

Symptoms

- Rheumatism—it has special affinity for small joints
- Severe drawing, erratic pain and stiffness in small joints, fingers, toes, ankle etc
- Shifting rheumatic pain, shifting from one part to another in every few minutes
- Cutting pain on closing hands
- Aching in wrists
- Shifting pain in limbs, in ankles, feet, toes causing a restless night

Symptoms *Worse*
- During menses
- In open air
- From coffee
- From motion

Symptoms *Better*
- From warmth
- Emission of flatus

- Weakness of knees when walking
- Rheumatoid arthritis especially in women
- Pain in muscles alternate with pain in joints
- Pain shifts from extremities to nape of neck
- Rheumatism worse during menses

The following symptoms generally accompany the above symptoms . . .

- Especially suited to women, during pregnancy, parturition, lactation
- Extraordinary *rigidity of os* causes delay of labour
- False labour pains. It revives labour pains and further progress of labour
- Habitual abortion from uterine debility
- Spasmodic pain in stomach
- Pains are intermittent, spasmodic and shifting in character
- Discoloration of skin, 'moth' spots on forehead, in women with menstrual and uterine disorders

If there is no improvement after one month then please consult a trained homoeopathic practitioner.

Acupressure

Generally this therapy offers effective relief from pain when administered by a trained practitioner.

Herbal Therapy

There are many herbs which decreases pain, stiffness and swelling, by blocking the inflammation. Choose from the following:

- *Curcumin extract*—400 gm three times daily. This is a *turmeric* extract, and has a powerful anti-inflammatory action
- *Ginger*—1-2 gm, three times daily, of powdered root, or make a tea from the fresh root, or cook
- *Chinese Skullcap (Scutellaria)*—2-4 gm three times daily. This has a highly potent anti-inflammatory and anti-oxidant effect
- *New Zealand Green-lipped Mussel*—350 mg, three times daily. This is a very effective herb. It is anti-inflammatory and also repairs the collagen part of cartilage
- 5 ml tincture made from 2 parts willow (salix spp) bark and 1 part each of black cohosh (cimicifuga racemosa) and nettle (urtica dioica), taken three times a day for relieving pain
- To relieve muscle tension, rub a tincture of lobelia (lobelia inflata) and cramp (viburnum opulus) bark on the affected area
- A poultice for swollen painful joint: mix two tablespoon *mullein* + two tablespoons *slippery elm* + one teaspoon *cayenne* + one teaspoon *lobelia*

Hydrotherapy

Swimming or other water exercises, preferably in a heated pool improves movement of affected joints and improves muscle strength. Shower for three minutes under very hot water followed by thirty seconds of cold water; this method improves circulation and skin function.

Yoga

Daily yoga practice may help loosen stiff, arthritis joints. Try the exercises shown here for painful joints:

- *Spider push-up* for joints of hand. Press your fingertips together firmly, holding your palms two to three inches apart. Then push your palms toward each other while keeping your fingertips touching and with your fingertips still together move them apart, relax, then repeat this 20 times *(See figure 3.2)*
- Thumb squeezer to ease stiff finger joints. Curl your fingers into a fist around your thumb, gently squeeze, then slowly release. Repeat this 10 times with each hand *(See figure 3.3)*
- *'C'* exercise—Do this exercise on your palms and knees in the table position; exhale and swing your head and buttocks as far to the left as you can. Breath deeply as you hold this position for 10 second, exhale as you slowly straighten your back, and then do the same movement to the right. Repeat this 10 times *(See figure 3.4)*
- *Dog* and *Cat*—The dog and cat helps to stretch your hips and back. Be on your palms and knees in the table position, inhale as you lower your back and lift your head and buttocks (Dog). Then exhale as you arch your back and drop your head and buttocks (Cat). Repeat it 10 times *(See figure 3.5)*

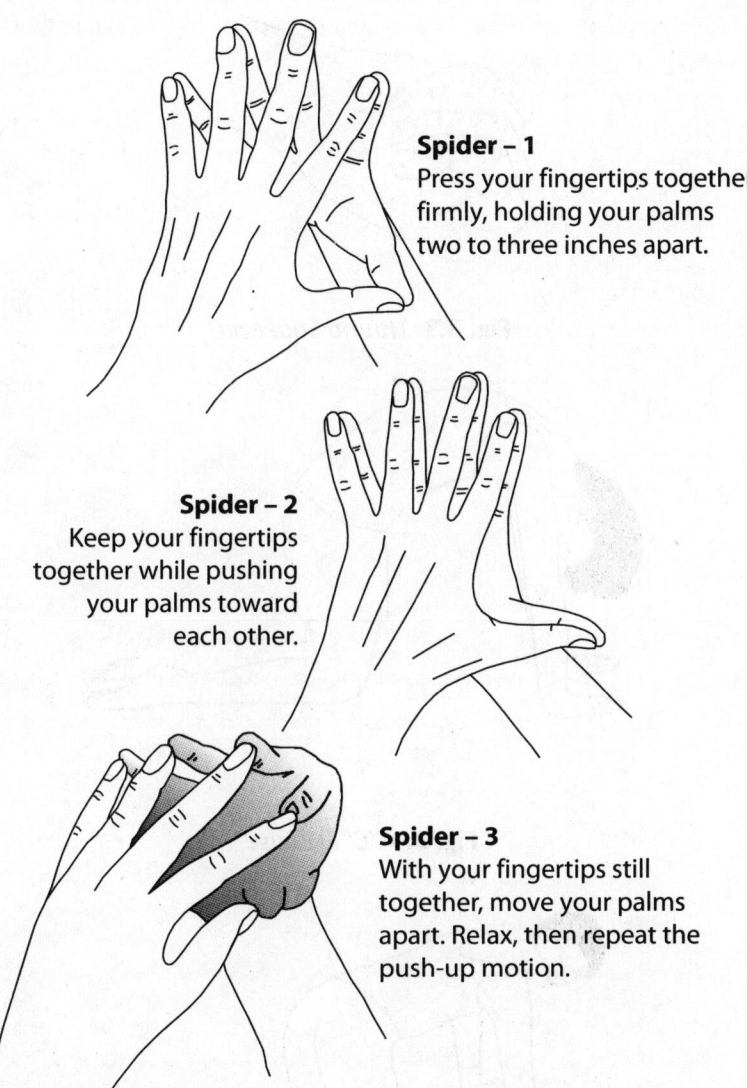

Fig. 3.2 *Spider Push-up*

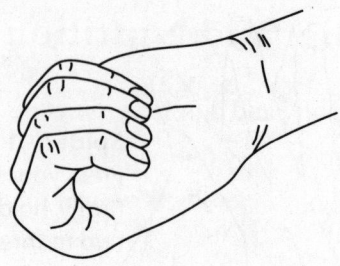

Fig. 3.3 *Thumb Squeezer*

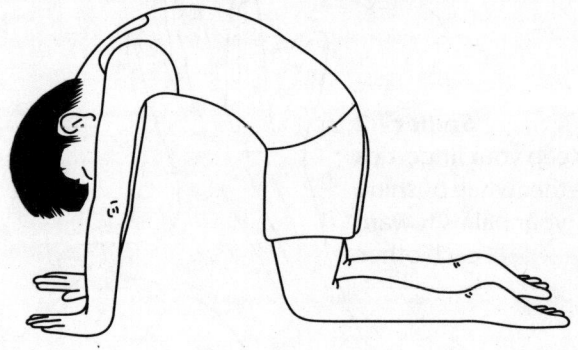

Fig. 3.4 *'C' Exercise*

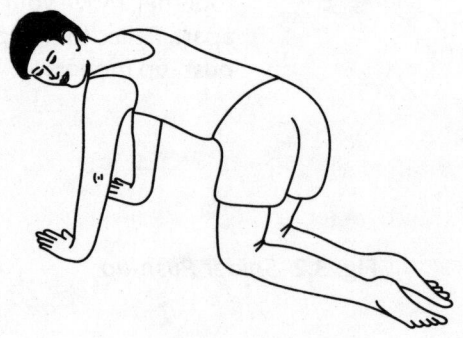

Fig. 3.5 *Dog and Cat*

Diet and Nutrition

- Avoid overeating and don't eat too quickly
- Chew everything very thoroughly
- Don't be anxious or stressed at meal time

What to eat

- All alkaline forming foods, which include generally all fruits and vegetables except pulses, asparagus, peas, broad beans, Brussels sprouts. Other alkaline forming foods are millet, yoghurt, fresh coconut, soya product and egg white
- Bananas, pineapples, apples and grapes
- Carrot, celery, beetroot, parsley, alfalfa, garlic, mushrooms
- Fruits—all berry fruits, blueberries, blackberries and cherries
- Sprouted grains, seeds and nuts
- Nuts and seeds, especially of sunflowers, sesame, walnuts, pumpkin seeds, almonds should be taken raw and fresh
- Grains—millet, rice, corn are the best. Use rye and oatmeal in moderation. Wheat causes many problems for many arthritis patients, so avoid it
- Have goat's milk or soya milk, egg and cottage cheese in moderation
- Oily fish
- Spirulina and wheat grass
- Turmeric and ginger
- Low-fat and low-protein vegetarian diet

What to reduce

- All acid-forming foods, especially meat and dairy products. Home made cottage cheese is fine. All these products increase inflammation
- Citrus fruits—sometimes the body does not metabolise these correctly
- Pulses

What to avoid

- Foods to which you are allergic. Use trial and error, preferably under the supervision of a homoeopathic physician
- Nightshade family: tomato, potato, pepper, capsicum, chilli
- All wheat flour, and everything made from it—bread, pasta, cereal and cakes
- Sugar and artificial sweeteners
- Added salt and hot spices
- All frozen and processed foods—cakes, cereals, jams, sausages etc
- Coffee, tea, cocoa, alcohol and soft drinks

Juice Therapy

- Raw and fresh, fruit and vegetable juices are of enormous benefit to a patient
- These must be freshly prepared and not canned or packed
- Dilute the juice and drink slowly
- They should not be mixed with hot liquids

Arthritis

- Beneficial juices:
  - Spinach and carrot
  - Carrot, ginger root, and apple
  - Cherry and blueberry
  - Pineapple
  - Broccoli, garlic clove and carrot
  - Pineapple, apple and ginger root
  - Parsley, broccoli, and spinach
  - Broccoli, lettuce and cabbage
  - Dark green vegetables

Home Remedies

- Hot fomentation and rest are very effective
- Hot fomentation from a heating pad or a hot bath or a hot water bottle wrapped in a towel
- Sea bathing has been found valuable
- Reduce weight if you are obese
- Warm coconut or mustard oil, mixed with two or three pieces of camphor should be massaged on stiff and painful joints
- Another massage oil—lavender + eucalyptus or camphor + ginger + rosemary. Mix all oils and put 15 drops of this oil to 30 ml of carrier oil (almond or avocado). A daily massage with this oil is beneficial for the patient
- Garlic may be taken raw or cooked
- Juice of one lime, diluted with water, may be taken once a day, preferably early in the morning

Chapter 4

Gout

A disturbance in the chemical balance of the body, in which chronic excess uric acid in the blood leads to deposition of needle-shaped urate crystal in and around joints and tendons, where they cause inflammation (gout is a form of arthritis). Gout is not a single disease. Gout not only causes inflammatory arthritis but also causes tendonitis, bursitis or cellulitis, tophaceous deposits, urolithiasis and renal disease.

The onset of Gout is sudden, unexpected, and excruciatingly painful. It strikes as an intense pain in a joint, most often the big toe, but sometimes other joints, including knees, elbows, thumbs or fingers. Generally, the pain disappears after medication, but it may recur.

Gout commonly occurs in middle aged men. Gout is uncommon in women and very rare in children. Men who are overweight or have high blood pressure are more prone to this disease.

Mild cases of gout may be controlled by diet alone. Chronic attacks of gout may require long-term treatment to prevent damage to the bone, cartilage and kidney. Chronic gout cases may have tiny, hard lumps accumulating in the soft flesh of the hands, feet, or earlobes. These deposits known as tophi are concentrations of uric acid crystals that can eventually cause aching, stiffness and protrusions.

Causes

- Hereditary
- Improper function of kidney which results in decreased excretion of urates in urine
- Reaction to alcohol
- Reaction to certain drugs, including antibiotics
- Enzyme deficiencies
- Lead poisoning
- Disorder is often associated with an injury or surgical procedure
- Highly proteinous diet
- Unidentified causes—Idiopathic causes
- Starvation—diminished renal excretion of uric acid
- Psoriasis—due to over production of uric acid
- Toxaemia of pregnancy—due to diminished excretion of uric acid
- May also occur in some cases of tumors or cancers

Gout

Symptoms

- Acute gout appears without warning
- Joint of a big toe is the site of the initial attack of gout in a majority of patients
- The joints of ankle, heel, knee and hand are also common sites (See figure 4.1)
- Sudden and intense pain in affected joint
- The gouty joint becomes hot, red, swollen and severely painful
- Acute attack may be accompanied by fever, anorexia, malaise, headache, nausea or a change in mood
- There is a tendency to have recurrent attacks, but symptoms typically do not last more than a week
- Acute gout attack is followed by deposition of tophi and secondary degenerative changes (See figure 4.2)

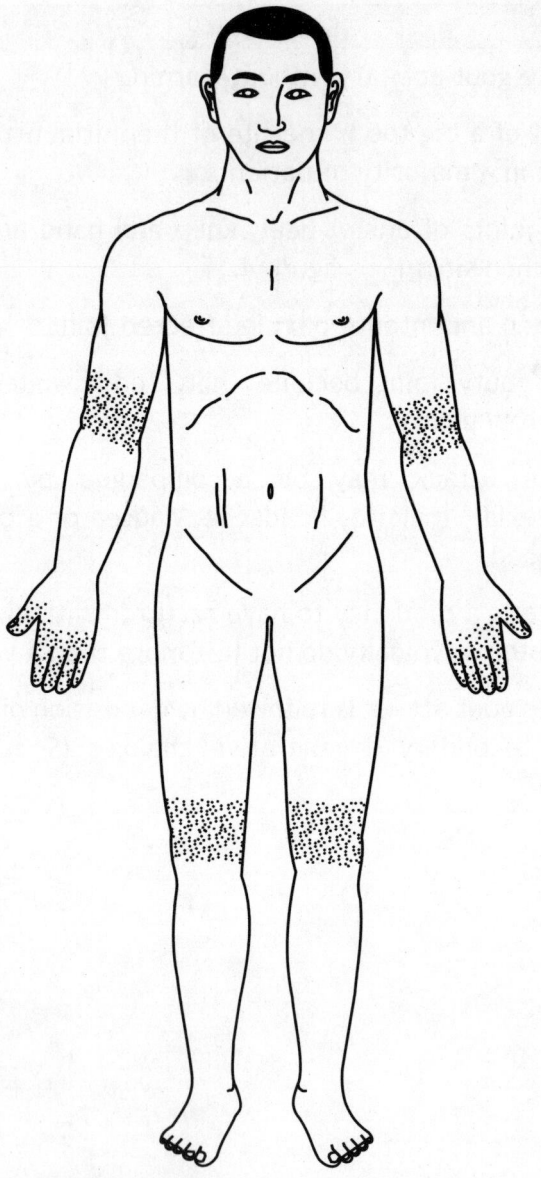

Fig. 4.1 *Gout can Also Affect Other Joints—Elbows, Hands and Knees. It May Affect Several Area at Once*

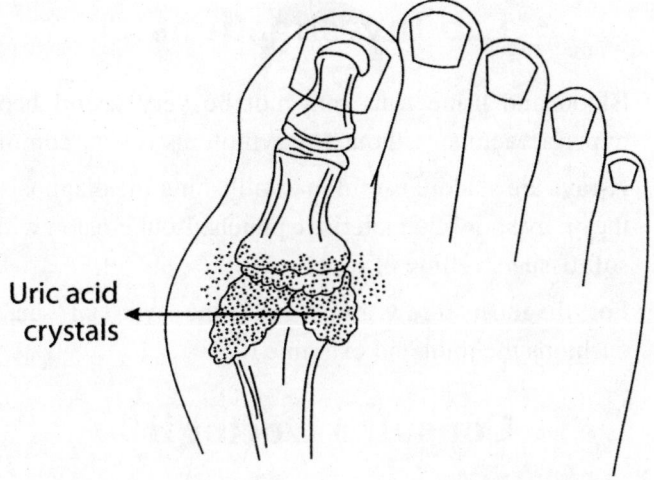

Joint with Gout

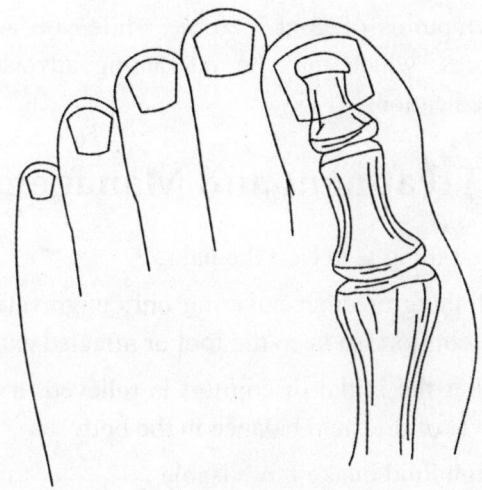

Normal Joint

Fig. 4.2 *Showing Crystals of Uric Acid Accumulated Between the Bones of Certain Joint, Most Commonly in Big Toe*

Lab Investigations

✦ Blood and urine tests may not be very useful because hyperuricaemia, without any symptoms is very common
✦ X-rays are seldom useful in establishing the diagnosis, but they may show characteristic punched-out erosion with the soft tissue swelling of tophi
✦ For diagnosis draw fluid from the synovial sac, that cushions the joint and examine it

Consult a Doctor if

✦ There is severe pain in a joint with sudden onset
✦ Pain lasts more than a day or recurs
✦ Pain is associated with chills and fever
✦ Symptoms of gout increase while you are taking some drugs, which may be interacting adversely with other medications

Treatment and Management

✦ First thing is to ease the pain
✦ Clothing or other covering only aggravates the pain and discomfort, so keep the foot or affected extremity, bare
✦ After the initial discomfort is relieved, try to control the level of uric acid balance in the body
✦ High fluid intake is advisable
✦ Reduce obesity if you are overweight
✦ All incidents of gout should be diagnosed and treated by a physician. If left untreated, uric acid deposits can eventually cause irreversible kidney damage

Homoeopathy

- Massage the area with Rhus tox. or Ruta ointment to relieve soreness and tenderness

The following remedies are commonly indicated in gout. Following is an analysis of overall signs and symptoms. You can take the remedies which cover maximum number of signs and symptoms that may relieve pain and other symptoms:

Ledum Palustre 30
4 pills three times daily for one month

Symptoms

- It is a very good remedy for *rheumatic* and *arthritic* affections in both acute and chronic form
- All the joints (like hips, knees, shoulders) are affected but especially small joints
- *Rheumatism begins in feet and travel upwards* and may even affect the heart
- Tearing, shooting, stinging and oppressive type of pain
- Throbbing in right shoulder
- Pressure in shoulder on raising or moving the arm
- Joint swollen, hot and pale without fever
- Cracking in joints
- Pain in right hip

Symptoms *Worse*
- At night
- From warmth of bed and bed covering
- From motion
- While walking
- From alcohol
- Towards evening

- Stiffness of knee with weakness and trembling when walking
- Trembling of hands on moving them or grasping anything
- *Soles painful*, can hardly step on them
- Ankles swollen
- *Gouty pains* shoot all through the foot and limbs and in joints
- Ball of great toe swollen
- Gout begins in lower limb and ascends
- Gouty deposits in wrists, fingers and toes
- Easy s*praining* of ankle
- Injured part feels cold or numb yet pains are better from cold application

Symptoms *Better*
• Cold application
• Putting feet in cold water
• From getting out of bed
• Rest
• In cool air
• From copious urination with red or pale deposits

The following symptoms generally accompany the above symptoms . . .
- There is a *general lack of animal heat,* feels chilly all the time
- Patient is irritable, desires to be alone
- The *parts affected are cold* to touch but not felt cold by the patient. He feels *better by cold application*
- Wounded parts are cold. Punctured wounds from nails or splinter and insect stings
- *Red pimples on forehead and cheeks*
- Anal fissures

- Severe bruises or black eye with discoloration of the area. Bruises that feel cold and numb

Bryonia Alba 30

4 pills three times daily for one month

Symptoms

- Joint red, hot, swollen with stitches and tearing
- Knees stiff and painful
- Every spot is painful on pressure
- During sprain and strain, joint is painful and swollen, distended with fluid with great stiffness
- Weariness and heaviness in all limbs and stiffness
- Swelling of elbow extending as far as middle of the upper arm and of forearm
- Swollen sensation in joints of finger on writing or taking hold of anything with pain
- Heaviness and weakness of legs while walking and on standing
- Stitching pain in hip joint extending to knees
- Weariness of thigh worse on ascending stairs, better while descending

Symptoms *Worse*

- From least motion and touch, caused by jar, by change of position, by any effort to talk, to cough, even by moving eye balls and by winking
- Hot weather after a cold spell and warmth
- Intolerance of heat
- After eating
- Exertion
- Suppressed perspiration
- 9 p.m.
- Morning

+ *Constant motion of left arm and leg*

The following symptoms generally accompany the above symptoms...

+ *Dryness of all mucous membranes* like lips, mouth, throat, nose, chest, digestive tract
+ *Excessive thirst.* Drinks large quantity of cold water
+ Symptom develop slowly
+ Patient is irritable
+ Patient wants to be left alone, wants to go home even when at home
+ Delirium—talks of business
+ Complaints which come on *after humiliation and anger*
+ Right-sided complaints
+ Physical weakness
+ Nausea and faintness when rising up
+ Pressure in stomach after eating, as of a stone
+ Bursting, splitting headache
+ Breast hot and painful, hard
+ Chest painful, while coughing
+ Constipation, stool *hard, dry, dark, as if burnt*
+ *Stitches* and stiffness in small of back
+ Cough, dry, spasmodic with gagging and vomiting, after eating and drinking

Symptoms *Better*
• Hard pressure and rest
• Lying on painful side
• From perspiring
• Cold things, cold air, cold water
• Darkened room

Acid Benzoicum 30

4 pills three times daily for one month

Symptoms

- ✦ Useful in persons with *uric acid diathesis*
- ✦ It is a useful remedy in *gouty cases,* use it when Colchicum fails
- ✦ Swelling of the wrist with gout deposits
- ✦ Gouty deposits, nodes are very painful. Nodes on joints of fingers and toes
- ✦ Tearing pain in great toe
- ✦ *Bunion* of great toe
- ✦ Joint cracks on motion
- ✦ Tearing pain in tendons and joints with stitches
- ✦ *Pain in tendo-achilles*
- ✦ Pain and swelling in knees
- ✦ Oedema of the lower extremities
- ✦ Pain changes position suddenly, metastasise with heart pain in the cardiac region
- ✦ Rheumatism and gout alternate with heart trouble with pain in cardiac region

Symptoms *Worse*
• In open air
• By uncovering
• Cold air
• Change in weather
• Motion
• Wine
• Urine scanty

Symptoms *Better*
• By heat
• Profuse urination

The following symptoms generally accompany the above symptoms . . .

- ✦ *Offensive odour* of urine accompanies all symptoms

- Urine is scanty, of a dark brown colour with repulsive odour; the smell exists at the time of urination and stays long afterwards
- Dribbling of urine in old men with enlarged prostate
- Renal insufficiency. Renal colic
- Rheumatism and gout alternate with heart trouble with palpitation and pain in cardiac region
- Stool offensive and liquid

Lithium Carbonicum 30

4 pills three times daily for one month

Symptoms

- Chronic rheumatism connected with heart lesions
- Rheumatic nodes
- Uric acid diathesis. It may cause gout
- Whole body is *sore*
- Rheumatic pains throughout shoulder joints, arms, fingers and small joints generally
- Joints swollen, red and painful on touch with itching around joints, better by hot water
- Pain in hollow of foot, extending to knee
- Ankle painful when walking
- Knees weak in the morning or on ascending stairs
- Nodular swelling in joints particularly joints of the fingers and the toes
- Paralytic stiffness all over body

Symptoms *Worse*
- In morning
- On right side

Symptoms *Better*
- On rising
- Moving about

Gout

The following symptoms generally accompany the above symptoms...

- Headache ceases while eating
- Nausea, acidity, *gnawing relieved by eating*
- Turbid urine, with mucus and red deposits
- Rheumatic soreness in heart region
- Patient cannot endure the slightest pressure from clothes, has palpitations and shocks about the heart
- In chronic cases, the patient's body increases in weight and becomes putty with clumsiness in walking and uneasiness in standing

Colchicum 30

4 pills three times daily for one month

Symptoms

- Very good remedy for *gout*
- Inflammation of big toe and heel
- Acute pain making patient scream when touched
- Tearing, stitching, jerking pains especially in finger joints
- Pains go from left to right
- Skin rose coloured, leaves a white spot under the pressure of the finger
- Metastasis from big toe to heart
- Shifting *rheumatism* present, generally small joint affected. *Pain shifting from one joint to another*

Symptoms *Better*

- From least touch and slightest motion, cannot bear to have it touched or moved
- Sundown to sunrise
- Motion
- Loss of sleep
- In autumn
- In evening
- Smell of food under preparation or strong odours
- Mental exertion
- Suppressed perspiration
- Cold, wet weather

- ✦ Joint stiff, feverish and tender and swollen
- ✦ Pains are shooting, tearing and twitches like electric shock
- ✦ Rheumatic pains all over the body— arms, back, neck and shoulder
- ✦ Swelling of the affected joint is red or pale with extreme tenderness

Symptoms *Better*
• Sitting
• Rest
• Stooping
• Rubbing
• Warmth
• From doubling up

- ✦ Sensation of pin and needles in hands and wrist, fingertips numb
- ✦ Tingling in finger nails
- ✦ Knee strike together, can hardly walk
- ✦ Oedematous swelling pits on pressure
- ✦ Pain in front of thigh
- ✦ Sharp pain down left arm
- ✦ Limbs weak, lame and tingling
- ✦ Cramps of calves

The following symptoms generally accompany the above symptom . . .

- ✦ There is always great prostration, internal coldness and tendency to collapse
- ✦ Violence of all symptoms, worse between sundown to sunrise
- ✦ *The smell of fluid causes nausea even to fainting;* he gags from mere mention of food especially fish, egg
- ✦ Great icy coldness in stomach
- ✦ Unquenchable thirst for cold drinks, alcoholic beverages

Gout

- Distension of abdomen, with gas, inability to stretch out legs
- Autumnal dysentery, stool shreddy and bloody

Lycopodium 30

4 pills three times daily for one month

Symptoms

- It is useful in chronic rheumatism and arthritis
- Rheumatic pain may occur in any of the joints of the body but knee and finger joints are commonly affected
- Numbness, drawing and tearing in limbs especially while at rest or at night
- Pain will often have started on right-side of body and moved over to left
- Spasmodic contraction and extension without pain
- Pains come and go suddenly
- Heaviness of arms
- Tearing in shoulder and elbow joints
- Tearing pain in joints with stiffness
- *Chronic gout,* with chalky deposits in joints with urinary trouble; red sand and clear urine

Symptoms *Worse*

- From right to left
- From above downwards
- 4 to 8 p.m.
- At night
- From heat or warm room
- Hot air
- Warmth of bed
- Warm application (expect throat and stomach which are better from warm drinks)
- On beginning to move

- Gout which affects especially the right side
- Pain in heel on treading as from a pebble
- Profuse sweat on the feet
- Hands and feet numb
- Swelling of feet, worse right side
- Cramps in calves and toes at night in bed
- Twitching and jerking

Symptoms *Better*
- From continued motion
- After midnight
- Stomach and throat complaint relieved by warm drink and food
- On getting cold
- In cool open air
- On being uncovered

The following symptoms generally accompany the above symptoms . . .

- In nearly all cases where Lycopodium is the remedy, some evidence of urinary or digestive disturbance will be found
- Ailment develops gradually
- A *right-sided* remedy, complaints travel from right to left or from above leading downwards
- Symptoms are generally *worse* from *4 p.m. to 8 p.m*
- Its patient is generally lean, flatulent with wrinkles and is *prematurely old*
- Carving for sweets and warm food and drinks
- Patient is *apprehensive, afraid to be alone,* spells or write wrong words
- Although *hungry but eating ever so little (few bites) create fullness*
- Food tastes sour

Gout

- Blisters on tongue
- Abdomen is bloated, full due to accumulation of wind, coupled with rumbling, gurgling and distension
- Stool hard, difficult to expel
- Dark, scanty urine, red sand in urine, frequency of urination increased at night
- Impotency in males

Mercurius Solubilis 30

4 pills two times daily for one month

Symptoms

- It is more effective in case of acute gout
- Joints sore, pale, swollen and occasional tearing pain
- Fingers flexed especially thumb with difficulty in opening
- Weakness of limbs, he can scarcely walk
- Lancinating pain in joints
- Drawing rheumatic pain in long bones particularly where the skin is thin, worse at night
- *Trembling in extremities, especially hands,* and jerking of arms
- Boring pain in periosteum of right tibia (leg bone) and drawing pain in tibia
- Swelling of feet and leg

Symptoms *Worse*

- At night
- Warmth of bed
- Warm room
- From lying on the right side
- Wet, damp weather
- Extreme of temperature
- Cold air, draft of air
- Sweating
- Daylight or firelight
- Before stool
- By sitting or walking
- During exercise

- Cold, clammy sweat on legs at night
- Tearing pain in hips and knees, worse open air
- Painful stiffness of wrist
- Rheumatic pain behind sternum, *cannot lie on right side*

Symptoms *Better*
• In moderate temperature
• From rest
• During the day

The following symptoms generally accompany the above symptoms . . .

- Complaints worse at night from change of weather, and warmth of bed. He is *sensitive to extremes of cold and heat*
- Glandular swelling with or without suppuration
- Profuse and offensive sweating with complaints; complaints worse with sweat
- Intense thirst for cold water, with moist mouth with excessive saliva, which he is constantly swallowing
- Discharges from all body increase and are offensive
- Fetid odour from mouth, metallic taste
- Body smells offensive
- Thick, moist coated tongue with imprint of teeth
- *Tremors* and trembling everywhere from least exertion
- Tension headache, *as if bandaged*
- Gums spongy and bleed easily with pain on chewing
- Dysentery *bloody, mucous stool* (more mucous than blood in stools), *with pain and tremors*
- Skin almost constantly moist with marked tendency for ulcers, boils and pus formation in general
- Emaciation with swelling of hand and feet with anaemia

Arnica Montana 30

4 pills three times daily for one month

Symptoms

- ✦ Rheumatism of muscular and tendinous tissue, especially of hip, back and shoulders
- ✦ It is suited to cases when any injury, however remote, seems to have caused the present trouble *After traumatic injury*
- ✦ A muscular tonic
- ✦ Limbs and body aches as if beaten joints as if sprained
- ✦ *Sore, lame and bruised feeling*
- ✦ Sharp, shooting, paralytic or sprained pains which quickly change place
- ✦ *Gouty affections.* Great fear at being touched or approached
- ✦ Sore, tender, red swelling of the joints in gout particularly of knee joint
- ✦ Gout with arthritic pains in the feet and the big toe as if sprained
- ✦ In arthritis especially hip joint is affected
- ✦ Rheumatism begins low down and works up
- ✦ Cannot walk erect, on account of bruised pain in pelvic region
- ✦ Paralytic pains in all joints during motion

Symptoms *Worse*
• Least touch
• Motion
• Rest
• Wine
• Damp cold
• Evening
• From speaking
• Blowing nose
• Almost any noise
• Lying on injured part
• From over-exertion
• Alcohol
• Old age

- ✦ Knee bends suddenly when walking, stitches when touched
- ✦ Twitching pain from left shoulder joint to middle finger
- ✦ Pain in back and limbs, as if bruised
- ✦ Deathly coldness of forearms
- ✦ Everything on which he is seems too hard
- ✦ Soreness after over-exertion
- ✦ Cracking in the right wrist when the hand is moved, as if dislocated
- ✦ During *Sprains* and *Strains* ligaments torn with swelling which is most prominent. Bruising and inflammation of the soft tissue around the joint
- ✦ When muscles or soft tissues are black and blue

Symptoms *Better*
• Lying down
• Lying with head low
• Warmth
• Rubbing and wrapping up warmly
• Long walk in cold weather
• Out stretched
• Changing position

Following symptoms generally accompany the above symptoms . . .

- ✦ Produces conditions similar to those resulting from injuries, falls, blows, contusions
- ✦ Especially suited to cases when any injury occurs. *After any traumatic injuries*
- ✦ Remote effects of injuries even though received years ago
- ✦ Whole body feels *sore and bruised, lame* and does not want to be approached, touched or jarred
- ✦ It *promotes healing,* reduces swelling, prevents pus formation
- ✦ It is very effective in bleeding of any kind

- *Head hot with cold body*
- Fetid breath
- Diarrhoea offensive and bloody
- *Violent spasmodic cough with facial herpes*
- Skin *black and blue*. Multiple small boils very painful. Acne characterised by *symmetry in distribution*
- *Aids recovery after an operation*

Calcarea Carbonica 30
4 pills three times daily for one month

Symptoms
- It is a useful remedy for rheumatoid arthritis, chronic and acute muscular rheumatism, gouty nodosities
- Rheumatic pains, after getting wet
- Sharp sticking pain, as if parts were sprained
- *Cold, damp feet,* feels as if damp stockings were worn
- Pains are shooting, cutting or tearing, sometimes confined to small spots
- Pains are associated with cramps, contraction, stiffness and weakness all over the body
- Cold knees
- Cramp in calves
- Sour foot sweat
- Swelling of joints, especially knee
- Inflammation of hip joints which is painfully sore

Symptoms *Worse*
- From exertion, mental or physical
- Ascending
- Cold in every form
- Washing, moist air, wet weather
- During full moon
- Standing
- After eating
- In the evening after midnight

- Burning of soles of feet which feel cold and dead at night
- Weakness in the muscles of thigh in morning, on beginning to walk, with stiffness, *worse with ascending stairs or any height*
- Pain in calves on stepping, on touch and on bending foot
- *Soles of feet raw*
- Ankles weary, feels as if dislocated
- Tearing in muscles
- Rheumatoid arthritis of finger joints with swelling and arthritic nodosities on hand and finger joints
- Pain in upper arm, as if beaten
- Sweating of palms of hands
- Sprained pain in right wrist, on motion
- Cramps in hands all night and trembling in afternoon, worse from lifting heavy weights

Symptoms *Better*
• Dry climate and weather
• Lying on painful side
• Sneezing
• Rubbing
• From drawing the limbs up
• While lying on the back in the dark and dry weather

The following symptoms generally accompany the above symptoms . . .

- It is generally suited to *children and women*
- The remedy is suited *to persons who are fatty, flabby and obese*
- Children whose head is too large, they *crave eggs and eat dirt,* and are prone to diarrhoea
- Children milestone are delayed especially walking and talking
- There is great sensitiveness to catch cold

- *Profuse perspiration,* local and general, from slight exertion; *while sleeping wetting the pillow*
- Patient is very *apprehensive, forgetful* and has a variety of fears
- Sensation of coldness in general of single parts—head, stomach and feet and legs
- Periodicity of symptoms—commonly of 7 to 14 days
- *Enlarged glands*—Tonsils and other glands
- *Nostrils sore* and *ulcerated*
- Sour taste in mouth
- Craving of *indigestible things—chalk, coal, pencils*
- Frequent sour eructations, sour vomiting. *All discharges sour*
- Dislike of fat. May be aversion to milk
- *Loss of appetite when overworked*
- Menses *too early, too profuse, too long* with vertigo. *Milky white discharge*
- Painless hoarseness, shortness of breath on walking especially on going upstairs
- Aversion to open air
- Fever with night sweats, especially on head

Causticum 30
4 pills three times daily for one month

Symptoms
- It is mainly useful in chronic rheumatic, arthritic and paralytic affections
- Generally indicated by tearing, drawing pains in the muscular and fibrous tissues, with deformities about the joints, especially knee and shoulder joints

- Restlessness in night with tearing pain of joints
- Pains are severe, generally remain in one joint for a long time
- Joints are stiff
- *Rheumatic tearing in limbs*
- Burning in joints
- Dull and tearing pain in hands and arm
- Rheumatism of the jaw with great stiffness
- Unsteadiness of *muscles of forearm* and hands
- Numbness, loss of sensation in hands
- Rheumatic pain of shoulders, cannot raise hand, painful stiffness between scapulae
- Pain in nape of neck as from bruises
- *Contracted tendons*
- Weak ankles, cannot walk without suffering
- Unsteady walking and easy falling
- *Restless legs at night*. Cannot find a position to lie still in bed for a moment at night
- Cracking and tension in knees, stiffness in hollow of knee
- Painful stiffness in the limbs through the hips, especially on rising from a seat or from a recumbent position

Symptoms *Worse*
- In dry cold wind
- In clear, fine weather
- Cold air
- From motion of carriage
- Expectoration
- Walking
- New moon
- After stools

Symptoms *Better*
- By warmth, especially heat of bed
- In damp, wet weather
- Open air
- Stooping low
- Emission of flatus

- Itching on the dorsum of feet

The following symptoms generally accompany the above symptoms . . .

- Causticum patient is sad, hopeless dark complexioned *intensely sympathetic*
- *Burning, rawness* and *soreness* are characteristic
- General tendency of paralytic affection
- Restlessness at night and faint-like sinking of strength. Thus weakness progresses towards paralysis
- Paralysis of single parts—vocal cords, muscles of swallowing, of tongue, eyelids, face, bladder and extremities
- Dirty white sallow skin with warts especially on the face
- Symptoms worse on right side of body
- *Coryza with hoarseness*
- *Pimples and warts* on nose
- Aversion to sweets
- Thirst for cold water but aversion to drinking
- Menses cease at night, *flow only during day*
- *Hoarseness* with pain in chest and *loss of voice*
- Cough with *raw soreness of chest*
- Expectoration scanty, must be swallowed
- Cough with *pain in hip*, worse in evening, *better with drinking cold water*
- Difficulty of voice of singers and public speakers
- *Warts* large, bleed easily, on tips of fingers and nose
- *Retention of urine*
- Bed wetting soon after falling asleep (during first sleep)

- Involuntary urine may also dribble while coughing or sneezing or after any excitement
- Constant mental stress, effects of shock or grief, any long standing worry

Sulphur 30
4 pills twice daily for fifteen days

Symptoms

- Rheumatic and arthritic complaints due to suppression of any skin disease
- *Painful stiffness* is main symptom, with or without effusion
- For preventing gouty diathesis there is no better remedy than *Sulphur*
- One of the leading remedy for synovitis
- *Hot, sweaty hands*
- Trembling of hands
- Sprained pain in wrist
- Pain in left shoulder as if joint is dislocated
- Jerking in deltoid
- Drawing pain in shoulder and arms
- Swelling in fingers in morning, sticking in tips at night; of flexure surface of right middle finger
- *Stoop shoulders*, cannot walk erect
- Tearing above the nail of left ring finger, worse in the evening

Symptoms *Worse*

- At rest
- Around 11 a.m.
- In morning
- Night
- Warmth of bed
- When standing
- Washing and bathing
- From alcoholic stimulants
- From weather changes
- Periodically

- ✦ Sharp drawing, shooting and stitches here and there
- ✦ Pains seem to ascend, is worse in mid-summer heat on clear and cloudless days
- ✦ Sweat in armpits, smelling like garlic
- ✦ Stiffness of knees and ankles
- ✦ *Burning in soles and hands at night*
- ✦ Weakness of thighs and legs
- ✦ Tearing extending into middle of thigh worse on standing and on ascending stairs
- ✦ Tearing through knee extending to feet when walking and sitting
- ✦ Sprained wrenching pain in joints with cracking and stiffness, particularly in knees and shoulders
- ✦ Sudden cramp-like, painful jerking about the hip joints with stiffness
- ✦ Tension, pain in joint on walking
- ✦ Tension in hollow of knees, as if too short, on stepping
- ✦ Inclination to cramp on stretching out feet
- ✦ Rheumatic gout with itching
- ✦ Swelling and inflammation of big toe with pain

Symptoms *Better*
• Dry, warm weather
• In open air
• Lying on right side
• From drawing up affected limbs

The following symptoms generally accompany the above symptoms . . .

- ✦ Burning everywhere in the body especially head, palm and sole
- ✦ *Dirty, filthy people,* prone to skin disease, dry and hard hair and skin

- Children—*cannot bear to be washed or bathed*
- Aversion on being washed
- *When carefully selected remedies fail to produce a favourable effect,* especially in acute diseases
- Itching eruption on the skin. Scratching is followed by burning
- *Standing is worse position* for patients, they cannot stand
- *Complaints are relapsing*—the patient seems to get almost well but the disease returns
- Redness of all orifices (lips, ears, eyelids, nostrils, anus, urethra etc.) as if pressed full of blood
- Discharges are offensive in character
- The discharges both of urine and faeces is painful to parts over which it passes; *parts around anus red, excoriated.* All the orifices of the body are very red
- *Milk disagrees,* craves sugar, sweets and fatty food
- *Great acidity* and sour eructations
- *Diarrhoea,* painless, *driving out of bed early in the morning*
- Weak, empty gone feeling and *faint about 11 a.m.*

Rhus Toxicodendron 30

4 pills three times daily for one month

Symptoms

- Hot, painful swelling of joint
- Tearing and drawing pain
- *Limbs stiff, paralysed sensation*
- Tenderness about knee joint
- Trembling after exertion
- Tingling in feet

- Loss of power in forearm and fingers
- Crawling sensation in the tips of finger
- *Tearing pain in tendons, ligament and tascture*
- Numbness after over work and exposure
- Soreness of condyles of bones
- Pains, aching, sore, bruised, tearing, shooting with heaviness, lameness and stiffness
- *Sprains, strains, torn ligaments and tendinitis*

Symptoms *Worse*
- The cold fresh air is not tolerable
- Damp weather and after rains
- From sitting and rising from sitting position or first attempt to move
- Approach of storms
- At night, especially in bed
- After overwork and exposure
- From gardening
- Checked perspiration
- Injuries after lifting and over-exertion

The following symptoms generally accompany the above symptoms . . .
- *Extreme restlessness* accompanies most symptoms. Cannot stay in one position, continued change of position
- Aching in bone with fever
- Tongue coated, except red triangular space at tip with great thirst
- Bitter taste in mouth
- Skin eruptions—red, swollen with intense itching
- Desire for milk
- Fever of typhoid character
- General or localised glandular swelling

- ✦ Trembling and palpitation of heart when siting still
- ✦ *Sensitive to open air,* putting the hand from under the bed-cover brings on cough

Calcarea Phosphorica 30

4 pills three times daily for one month

Symptoms

- ✦ Shooting, tearing and aching type of rheumatic pain in all parts of body especially knees, loins and thumb
- ✦ Pain with stiffness, coldness, *numbness and crawling sensation*
- ✦ Pain becomes worse by any change of weather
- ✦ Buttocks, back and limbs fall asleep
- ✦ Weary when going upstairs. Cannot rise from seat. Staggering in old people when rising from a seat
- ✦ Pain in joints and bones excited or increased by every draft of cold damp air
- ✦ Rheumatism of cold weather, getting well in spring and returning in autumn

Symptoms *Better*
• From external heat
• Warm compresses
• From warmth of bed
• Continued movement
• Change of position
• Moving affected partly
• Rubbing
• From stretching out limbs

The following symptoms generally accompany the above symptom . . .

- ✦ For anaemic persons, especially *anaemic children* who are flabby, have cold extremities and feeble digestion

- Children—*emaciated, unable to stand, and slow in learning to walk*
- *Feels complaints more when thinking about them*
- *Numbness and crawling* are characteristic sensations
- Symptoms get worse by wet cold air and every *change of weather*
- Headache, *worse near the region of sutures*
- Glandular enlargement—swollen tonsils. *Adenoid growths*
- *Craving for bacon, ham, salted or smoked meat*
- *Much flatulence.* Flatulence temporarily relieved by sour eructation
- Pain in abdomen *at every attempt to eat*
- Diarrhoea from juicy fruits, during dentition *with fetid flatus*
- White discharge in females, *like white of egg*

Symptoms *Worse*

- Exposure to cold and damp weather
- Cold air
- Melting snow
- Changeable weather
- East winds
- Mental exertion
- Dinner
- After a meal, especially juicy fruits
- Motion

Symptoms *Better*

- In summer
- Warm, dry atmosphere
- Lying down
- Rest
- Passing wind

Formica Ruta 30

4 pills three times daily for one month

Symptoms

- Mainly an arthritic remedy
- Right side most commonly affected
- Chronic gout and stiffness in joints
- Sometimes acute attack of gout pain; pain worse with motion; pain better with pressure
- Rheumatic pain—stiff and contracted joints
- *Rheumatic complaints come suddenly with restlessness; sweat does not relieve any complaints*
- Muscles feel strained and torn from their attachments
- Complaints from over lifting
- *Weakness of lower extremities*
- Pain in hips
- Paralysis of all limbs

Symptoms Worse
- Cold and cold washing
- Dampness
- Before a snowstorm
- Right side
- Motion
- Sitting

Symptoms Better
- Warmth
- Pressure
- Rubbing
- After midnight
- Combing hair

The following symptoms generally accompany the above symptoms . . .

- Cracking in left ear with headache
- Coryza and stopped-up feeling in nose
- It has marked deterrent influence on the formation of polypi

Gout

- Pain in bowels before stool
- Drawing pain around navel before stool
- Skin—red, itching and burning
- Nodes around joints
- Profuse sweat without relief

Pulsatilla 30

4 pills three times daily for one month

Symptoms

- Drawing, tearing pains in joints with swelling and redness especially hips, knees, elbows and small joints of hand and feet
- The *pains shift* rapidly *from one part to another*
- Can hardly give symptoms and starts crying
- Rheumatic pains are so severe that the patient is compelled to move slowly, as easy motion relieves the pain
- Drawing, tensive pain in thighs and legs with restlessness and *chilliness*
- *Pain in limbs*, tensive pain, *letting up with a snap*
- Pain appears in a part, increase to a climax and then disappear suddenly from the part
- Pain in limbs in the morning in bed on waking with stiffness

Symptoms Worse

- From heat
- Rich fat food
- After eating
- In warm close room
- Evening
- At twilight
- Lying on left or on painless side
- When allowing feet to hand down
- At beginning to move
- On being seated or flexing (back)

- Hip-joint painful
- Knees swollen, with tearing, drawing pains
- Boring pain in heels like pricking of nails towards evening, *suffering worse from letting the affected limb hang down*
- Feet red inflamed and swollen
- Numbness around elbow
- Tearing in the shoulder joint obliging him to bend arms, extends intermittently to wrists and fingers
- Legs feel heavy and weary
- Nervousness, intensely felt about the ankles

Symptoms *Better*
• Cool open air
• Slow motion
• Cold application
• Cold food and drink
• Lying on painful side
• Pressure or tying up tightly especially in head
• Rest

The following symptoms generally accompany the above symptoms . . .

- Very often indicated in the later, established stage of illness
- It is pre-eminently a female remedy, especially for mild gentle, sad, crying, readily *weeps while talking, changeable,* contradictory
- Feels better by consolation
- The patient is chilly but she *feels better in open air and seeks the open air*
- Dry mouth but absence of thirst with nearly all complaints
- *Secretion* from all mucous membranes are *thick, bland and yellowish-green*
- *Symptoms ever changing*—no two stools, no two attacks alike; very well one hour, very miserable the next

- Pains *rapidly shifting* from one part to another
- Eyes inflamed and agglutinated
- Cracks in middle of lower lips. *Yellow or white tongue*, covered with a tenacious mucous
- Desire for rich and fatty food, which leads to indigestion
- Dry cough in the evening and at night, must sit up in bed to get relief and loose cough in the morning. Pressure upon the chest and soreness
- Menses too late, scanty or suppressed
- Useful remedy to begin the treatment in a chronic case

Staphysagria 30
4 pills three times daily for one month

Symptoms
- Arthritic nodosities of joint, especially of the fingers
- Inflammation of phalanges with sweating and suppuration
- Stiffness and sense of fatigue in all joints
- Muscles, especially of calves, feel bruised
- Debilitated all over joints after walking, mainly shoulder, sacral and hip joints
- Sprained pain in right shoulder when walking
- Extremities feel beaten, as after a long walk, and painful
- Stiffness of joints in morning, on rising in bed

Symptoms *Worse*
• Least touch on the affected part
• From anger
• Indignation
• Grief
• Loss of vital fluids
• Sexual excesses
• Tobacco

- ✦ Sticking in right knee in morning, worse motion, changing on touch to pain
- ✦ Jerking in muscle of thumb, worse tip

Symptoms *Better*
• From warmth
• Rest at night
• After breakfast

- ✦ Itching and burning on left thumb
- ✦ Paralytic drawing in finger joints, worse motion
- ✦ Paralytic pain in bones, worse with motion and touch, especially left upper arm
- ✦ Oppressive drawing all over worse with touch
- ✦ Dull aching pain extending to hip joint and small of back

The following symptoms generally accompany the above symptoms . . .

- ✦ Nervous affection with marked irritability
- ✦ Effect of sexual excess or dwelling too much on sexual object
- ✦ *Very sensitive,* least action or harmless words offend
- ✦ Ailment from chagrin or offended pride, anger, grief
- ✦ *Violent outburst of passion*
- ✦ Child cries for many things, after receiving, they refuse or throw away
- ✦ *Craving for tobacco*
- ✦ Extreme hunger even when stomach is full
- ✦ *Recurrent styes, chalazae on eyelids* especially upper lid
- ✦ Toothache during menses
- ✦ *Teeth black and crumbing,* decay on edges
- ✦ *Stitches in throat, flying to the ear on swallowing,* especially left side
- ✦ Pain in abdomen after an abdominal operation

Gout

- *Irritable bladder in young married women,* ineffectual urging to urinate
- Intolerable urging to urinate, pain after urination and burning with prostatic enlargement
- *Sensation as if drops of urine were rolling continuously along the channel*
- Eczema of head, ear, face and body; thick scabs, dry and violent itching
- *Scratching in one place, after itching ceases, it appears in another part.*

Aconite Napellus 30

4 pills three times daily for one month

Symptoms

- It is useful in sudden onset of an *acute rheumatism* and *acute arthritis*
- Sudden onset of disease with fever
- *Numbness and tingling*, shooting pains, icy coldness and insensibility of hands and feet
- Bruised feeling over entire body
- Heaviness of all limbs
- Arms feel lame bruised, heavy, numb
- Pain down left arm
- *Hot hands* and *cold feet*

Symptoms *Worse*

- In evening and night about midnight
- In warm room
- Lying on affected side
- From severe cold weather and dry cold winds
- From music
- From intense heat especially sun's heat
- Hot days and cold night
- Warm covering
- From tobacco-smoke

- Swelling of hands
- Numbness and tingling in finger
- Rheumatic inflammation of joints, red shining swelling, very sensitive to contact
- Weak and lax ligaments of all joints
- Painless cracking of all joints
- Hip joint and thigh feels lame, especially after lying down
- Knees unsteady, disposition of foot to turn
- Sensation as if drops of water trickled down the thigh
- Rheumatism with fever; fever high grade with restlessness, fear and anxiety of mind and nervous excitability. He is unappeasable, tossing about with agony, skin hot and dry but sweat drenching on parts laid on
- *Bright red hypothenar eminence on both hands*

Symptoms *Better*
• Open air
• Rest
• By uncovering
• Sitting still
• After perspiration

The following symptoms generally accompany the above symptoms . . .

- *Physical and mental restlessness* is the most characteristic symptom of Aconite
- *Acute and sudden onset and violent invasion, with fever*
- *Complaints and tension* caused by exposure to dry *cold weather*, draught of cold air, checked perspiration and also from very *hot weather*
- Great *fear, anxiety* and worry accompany every ailment
- *Fear of death, fear the future*
- Its action is brief and *shows no marked periodicity*
- Burning thirst—for large quantity
- *Heavy,* pulsating, *hot, bursting* headache

- Vertigo, *worse on rising*
- Very sensitive to light, music, smell, touch and pain
- Burning in internal parts, *tingling, numbness and coldness*
- Tongue coated white
- Vomiting, with fever, heat, profuse sweat and increased urination
- Urine scanty, red, hot and painful
- *Oppressed breathing* on least motion. *Hoarse, dry, croupy cough*
- Shortness of breath, cough worse *at night* and *after midnight*
- *Palpitation with anxiety* and tingling in finger
- Fever with *great thirst* for cold water and *restlessness*. Cold waves passes through him
- Most complaints disappear when sitting still

Cinchona Officinalis 30
4 pills three times daily for one month

Symptoms
- It is more useful in chronic cases of gout and rheumatism
- *Pain in limbs and joints,* as if sprained, *worse with slight touch* and better by hard pressure
- Joint swollen and very sensitive with dread of open air
- Drawing and tearing pain in every joint
- Tendency of limbs to go to sleep
- Weakness of joints worse in the morning and when sitting
- Paralytic jerking and tearing in long bones, worse with touch
- Pain in thigh bone as if periosteum had been scraped with a dull knife

- Sensation as if there is a string around the limb
- Great debility, trembling and numb sensation
- Knees give a way while walking, worse with ascending stairs
- Hot swelling of right knee with pain extending to thigh and leg
- Aversion to exercise and sensitive to touch
- Chronic synovitis of the knee
- In case of chronic gout when it is monoarticular form and also intervals between attacks
- One hand icy cold and other hand warm

Symptoms *Worse*
- Slightest touch
- After eating
- At night
- Drafts of air
- Every other day
- Prolonged exertion
- Motion
- Loss of vital fluids
- Bending over
- From walking which makes him dizzy
- From fruits and Milk
- From perspiration

The following symptoms generally accompany the above symptoms . . .

- Ailments *from loss of vital fluids,* especially haemorrhages, excessive lactation, diarrhoea
- Symptoms with *marked periodicity,* return every other day, or regularly in season at same time
- Rapid general weakness with tendency of sweating from least excretion as well as sleep
- Patient is disobedient, depressed and ready to offend others
- Excessive *sensitivity to light, touch* but relief from hard pressure on painful part
- Throbbing headache, as if the skull would burst

- ✦ Excessive flatulence of stomach and bowels, belching gives no relief. Abdomen swollen like a drum with gas
- ✦ Frothy, watery, undigested stool; *painless diarrhoea*
- ✦ Passive haemorrhage from all outlet of the body with dark clotted blood
- ✦ *Intermittent fever worse every other day,* no thirst during heat, great thirst during sweat
- ✦ Anaemia and loss of appetite

Symptoms *Better*
• By bending double
• Hard pressure
• Warmth
• Open air
• Loose clothing
• Lying down

Guaiacum φ

10 drops (mix with water) two times daily for one month

Symptoms

- ✦ Its main action is on fibrous tissue, that is why adopted to arthritic and rheumatic complaints.
- ✦ It is very valuable in *acute rheumatism*
- ✦ Rheumatic pain in shoulders, arms and hands
- ✦ Joints swollen, painful and intolerant of pressure, cannot bear heat
- ✦ Stinging pain in limbs
- ✦ Arthritic lancination followed by contraction of limbs

Symptoms *Worse*
• Heat
• From motion
• Cold wet weather
• Pressure
• Touch
• From 6 p.m. to 4 a.m.
• When sitting
• In the morning immediately on rising
• In evening before sleep

- *A feeling of heat* in the affected limbs
- Gouty tearing with contraction. Immovable stiffness

Symptoms *Better*
• External pressure

- *Gouty and rheumatic pain in head* and face, *extending to neck*
- Ankle pain extending up the leg, causing lameness
- Contraction of limbs, stiffness and immobility. Feeling that he must stretch
- *Growing pains*
- Aching in bones
- *Stiff neck and sore shoulder*

Following symptoms generally accompany the above symptoms . . .

- It has *free foul secretions* and *unclean odour* from *whole body*
- Promotes suppuration of abscess
- *Acute tonsillitis.* Throat dry and burn
- *Desire for apples* and other fruits. Aversion to milk
- Patient feels as if his eyes are swollen and protruded and the lids appear too short to cover them
- *Feels suffocated*

Magnesia Phosphorica 30

4 tablets three times daily for one month

Symptoms

- Neuralgic pain and cramping of muscles
- In sprain and strain sharp, stabbing, shooting pain

- ✦ Pain generally sharp, cutting, piercing, knife like stabbing, shooting, stitching, lightening like
- ✦ Involuntary shaking of hands
- ✦ Cramps in calves
- ✦ Writer's and player's cramp
- ✦ Weakness in arms and legs
- ✦ Finger tips numb and stiff
- ✦ General muscular weakness

Symptoms *Worse*
• On the right side
• Touch
• Night
• Cold bathing or washing
• Being uncovered
• Walking in fresh air

The following symptoms generally accompany the above symptoms . . .

- ✦ Suitable for lean, thin emaciated persons who are forgetful, easily tired, drowsy, averse to mental effort
- ✦ Main remedy for *spasmodic pain; pain generally sudden and severe*
- ✦ Painful ailment relieved by the *application of heat*
- ✦ Pain shifts rapidly and usually affects the right side of the body
- ✦ Craving for sugar, averse to coffee
- ✦ May have thirst for cold drinks
- ✦ *Menstrual cramping* better after the flow begins
- ✦ Indicated for *all forms of cramp*, spasmodic and neuralgic pains in head, face, teeth, abdomen or stomach
- ✦ A five remedy for the tummy pains of babies

Symptoms *Better*
• Warmth and heat
• Bending double
• Pressure
• Friction

- ✦ Flatulent colic, forcing the patient to bend double, accompanied with belching of gas, which gives no relief. Bloated abdomen, must loosen cloth, walk about and constantly pass flatus
- ✦ Spasmodic cough, whooping cough
- ✦ Angia pectoris
- ✦ In fever, chills run up and down the back with shivering
- ✦ Great dread of cold air, *of uncovering,* of touching affected part, of cold bathing or walking, of moving

Caulophyllum 30

4 pills three times daily for one month or Caulophyllum mother tincture, 15 drops in luke warm water two times daily for one month.

Symptoms

- ✦ Rheumatism—it has special affinity for small joints
- ✦ Severe drawing, erratic pain and stiffness in small joints, fingers, toes, ankle etc
- ✦ Shifting rheumatic pain, shifting from one part to another in every few minutes
- ✦ Cutting pain on closing hands
- ✦ Aching in wrists
- ✦ Shifting pain in limbs, in ankles, feet, toes causing a restless night
- ✦ Weakness of knees when walking

Symptoms *Worse*
• During menses
• In open air
• From coffee
• From motion

Symptoms *Better*
• From warmth
• Emission of flatus

- Rheumatoid arthritis especially in women
- Pain in muscles alternate with pain in joints
- Pain shifts from extremities to nape of neck
- Rheumatism worse during menses

The following symptoms generally accompany the above symptoms . . .

- Especially suited to women, during pregnancy, parturition, lactation
- Extraordinary *rigidity of os* causes delay of labour
- False labour pains. It revives labour pains and further progress of labour
- Habitual abortion from uterine debility
- Spasmodic pain in stomach
- Pains are intermittent, spasmodic and shifting in character
- Discoloration of skin, 'moth' spots on forehead, in women with menstrual and uterine disorders

If there is no improvement after taking the above remedies then please consult a trained homoeopathic practitioner.

Acupressure

Acupressure points for relieving the pain of a gouty toe are several locations on the affected joint itself, among them: Spleen 3 *(figure 4.3)*, at the side of the metatarsal joint behind the big toe; Stomach 4 *(figure 4.4)*, at the centre of the top of the instep; and Liver 2 *(figure 4.5)*, just behind the space between the big and second toes. Press each of these points firmly for 60 seconds.

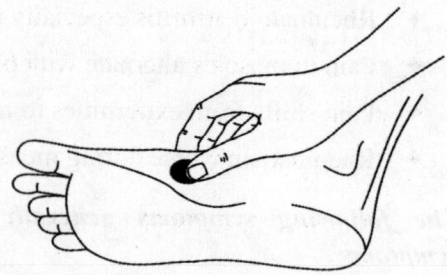

Fig. 4.3 *Spleen 3*

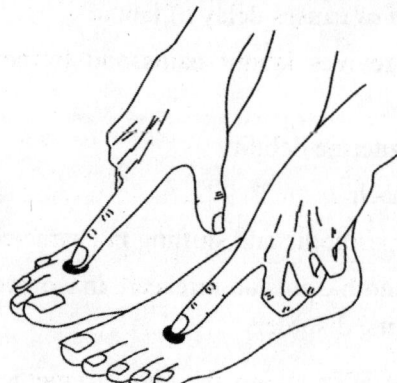

Fig. 4.4 *Stomach 4*

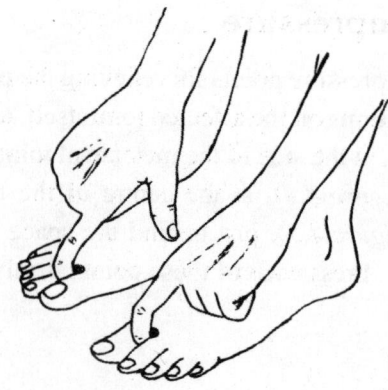

Fig. 4.5 *Liver 2*

Herbal Therapy

+ Drink an infusion of 2 tsp celery seed or grave root (Eupatorium purpureum) in a cup of water, three times a day
+ 10-15 drops of colchicum tincture three times daily. This herb prevents inflammation
+ Wild carrot, juniper, buck-bean, guaiacum and willow are all specific to gout.

Diet and Nutrition

Dietary regimens are necessary for preventing attacks of gout on people showing a hereditary predisposition.

What to eat . . .

+ Low protein diet. A vegetarian diet is good
+ Lots of vegetables, *garlic* dissolves uric acid. A high complex carbohydrate diet increases the excretion of uric acid
+ Whole grain such as brown rice, millet, corn, oat and rye
+ High levels of water, juices and herbal tea, because they help to dilute urine and promote excretion of uric acid
+ Small amount of nuts, pulses and seeds
+ High potassium foods—dried fruits, banana, mango, potato and tomatoes
+ Red sour cherries and all berry fruits. Even canned cherries are beneficial, if fresh ones are out of season
+ Pineapple

What to reduce . . .

+ Limit your wheat intake

- Pulses are rich source of protein, so eat them only twice in a week
- Meat, dairy products, eggs, poultry and fish. Avoid them totally during an attack
- Asparagus, mushrooms, spinach and green leafy vegetables
- Fruits, as it increases sugar

What to avoid . . .

- All glandular meats, red meat and meat extracts such as bouillon and gravies; organ meats such as liver, sweet breads, and kidney
- Shellfish and certain kinds of preserved fish, including sardines, herring, and anchovies, as their purine levels are very high
- Yeast
- Salt and spices
- Sugar and refined flour and everything made with them
- Gelatin, as it forms uric acid
- Alcohol, coffee, tea and soft drinks. Beer particularly high in purines
- Fats
- Overeating

Juice Therapy

- Cherries and strawberries juice
- Wheat grass, mint sprigs and pineapple juice
- Apple and celery juice
- Apple and strawberries juice
- Parsley, spinach, carrot and apple juice
- Fresh pineapple juice.

Reflexology

A reflexology practitioner will massage the appropriate area at the centre of the sole of foot, which helps to restore balance to the kidneys and spleen, the organs responsible for uric acid production.

Home Remedies

The first concern in an attack of gout is to reduce pain and inflammation

- Apply a plastic bag containing a few ice cubes to the joint, this will help in relieving pain and swelling. Wrap the cold bag in a soft cloth or towel and hold it against the painful area for upto five minutes at a time, then repeat it
- Hot epsom salt baths increase the elimination of uric acid through the skin. About 250-500 gm of these salt may be added to tolerably hot water and soak for 20 minutes just before bedtime
- Fresh air and outdoor exercise are also necessary
- Patient should eliminate as much stress from his life as possible
- Some home remedies are:
  - *Cherry*—The patient should consume about fifteen to twenty five cherries a day, after some time it reduces to 10 cherries a day
  - *French bean*—French or string bean juice should be taken daily
  - *Banana*—A diet of banana only for three or four days is advised. A patient can take 8 or 9 banana daily during this period and nothing else

- *Lime*—A juice of half a lime with a glass of water, should be taken twice daily
- *Apple*—The patient is advised to take one apple after each meal.

Prevention

+ If gout runs in the family, one should moderate their intake of alcohol, fats and high-purine food, and should keep their weight under control
+ Blood and urine tests during routine checkup are advisable

CHAPTER 5

Bursitis

Inflammation of bursa is known as bursitis. Whenever your bones, tendons, and ligaments move against each other, particularly near joints, the points of contact are cushioned by small fluid-filled sacs called *bursae*. More than 150 bursae in your body helps joint to operate smoothly by reducing friction.

Bursitis may develop at the site of persistent or recurrent pressure (for example housemaid's knee, students' elbow, coachman's bottom, tailor's ankle, bunion), or when a joint is overused, but often occurs without any obvious reason. The inflammation of the bursa results in the effusion of a clear fluid within the sac, causing pressure on surrounding tissues. The immediate signal is pain with swelling and tenderness. Prolonged inflammation causes the bursal sac to thicken and may cause pressure erosion on the adjacent bones. Chronic bursitis when left untreated can lead to the formation of calcium deposits, normally in soft tissues, sometime causing permanent immobilisation of the affected joint.

Shoulder has the greatest range of motion of all the joints in the body and is the most common site for bursitis. The pain is generally felt on top of the shoulder. Pain generally increases during sleep at night and decreases by normal activity of joint. Elbow, hips and knees are also prone to bursitis.

Causes

- Generally caused by excessive pressure or friction over the bursae
- An injury
- The cause of soreness of shoulder in professional and amateur athletes is due to bursitis, which comes from running, throwing, and jumping or the exaggerated arm swing used in tennis, baseball and bowling
- Working for extended periods in usual positions can also bring on a bursitic attack
- Heavy weight lifting also causes bursitis
- Sometimes a bursa may get infected by an infection. It occurs commonly in trochanteric bursa or prepatellar bursa
- Aspiration distinguishes friction bursitis from infective suppurative bursitis

Symptoms

- Pain, inflammation, swelling and tenderness in joint particularly during stretching or extension when lifting, exercising
- Restriction of movement of the joint

Consult a Doctor if

✦ Pain in the joint persists for more than a few days; you may be experiencing a strained ligament tendon, or the onset of arthritis

✦ Swelling persists after taking a pain killer drug

Treatment and Management

Bursitis generally disappears in a few days or weeks, but you must take precaution to avoid further strain or injury. It can be treated by rest of the affected joint.

After any injury immediate medical attention is very important. The RICE approach should be followed: Rest the injured area. Ice should be applied to the injured area. Compress the area with an elastic bandage. Elevate the injured body part above heart level.

Homoeopathy

The following remedies are commonly used in bursitis:

Arnica Montana 30
4 pills three times daily for one month

Symptoms

✦ Rheumatism of muscular and tendinous tissue, especially of hip, back and shoulders

✦ It is suited to cases when any injury, however remote, seems to have caused the present trouble *After traumatic injury*

✦ A muscular tonic

✦ Limbs and body aches as if beaten; joints as if sprained

- *Sore, lame and bruised feeling*
- Sharp, shooting, paralytic or sprained pains which quickly changes place
- *Gouty affections.* Great fear at being touched or approached
- Sore, tender, red swelling of the joints in gout particularly of knee joint
- Gout with arthritic pains in the feet and the big toe as if sprained
- In arthritis especially hip joint is affected
- Rheumatism begins low down and work up
- Cannot walk erect, on account of bruised pain on pelvic region
- Paralytic pains in all joints during motion
- Knee bends suddenly when walking, stitches and touched
- Twitching pain from left shoulder joint to middle finger
- Pain in back and limbs, as if bruised
- Deathly coldness of forearms
- Everything on which he lies seems too hard
- Soreness after over-exertion

Symptoms *Worse*
- Least touch
- Motion
- Rest
- Wine
- Damp cold
- Evening
- From speaking
- Blowing nose
- Almost any noise
- Lying on injured part
- From over excretion
- Alcohol
- Old age

Symptoms *Better*
- Lying down
- Lying with head low
- Warmth
- Rubbing and wrapping up warmly
- Long walk in cold weather
- Out stretched
- Changing position

- Cracking in the right wrist when the hand is moved, as if dislocated
- During *Sprains* and *Strains* ligaments torn with swelling which is most prominent. Bruising and inflammation of the soft tissue around the joint
- When muscles or soft tissues are black and blue

Following symptoms generally accompany the above symptoms . . .

- Produces conditions similar to those resulting from injuries, falls, blows, contusions
- Especially suited to cases when any injury occurs; *After any traumatic injuries*
- Remote effects of injuries even though received years ago
- Whole body feels *sore and bruised, lame* and does not want to be approached, touched or jarred
- It *promotes healing,* reduces swelling, prevents pus formation
- It is very effective in bleeding of any kind
- *Head hot with cold body*
- Fetid breath
- Diarrhoea offensive and bloody
- *Violent spasmodic cough with facial herpes*
- Skin *black and blue*. Multiple small boils very painful. Acne characterised by *symmetry in distribution*
- *Aids recovery after an operation*

Phytolacca 30

4 pills three times daily for one month

Symptoms

- It mainly acts well in chronic rheumatism
- A sore, bruised, aching feeling all over body; he feels he must move, movement increases his pain and soreness
- Rheumatic pain, worse in the morning
- *Pains fly like electric shocks*
- Shooting, lancinating pain shifting rapidly
- Rheumatic swelling are hard, painful on touch and intensely hot
- Shooting pain in cardiac region alternating with pain in right shoulder
- Shooting pain in right shoulder, with stiffness and inability to raise arm
- Pain on undersides of thighs
- *Aching of heels,* relieved by elevating feet
- Pain in right knee in afternoon, worse in open air and damp weather
- Pain in legs, patient dreads to get up and move

Symptoms *Worse*

- In the morning on rising
- Sensitive to electric changes
- Effects of a wetting, when it rains
- Exposure to damp, cold weather
- Night
- Motion
- Right side
- Hot drinks (especially in throat problem)

Symptoms *Better*

- Warmth
- Dry weather
- Rest

Bursitis

- Pain like shocks
- Swelling in feet
- Pain in ankle and feet
- Neuralgic pain in big toes
- Rheumatism of fibrous and periosteal tissue

The following symptoms generally accompany the above symptoms . . .

- Aching, soreness, restlessness, weakness are guiding general symptoms
- Glandular swelling with heat and inflammation
- *Pain flying like electric shocks;* rapidly shifting pains
- *Increased secretion of tears*
- Right-sided remedy especially in throat
- *Children bite teeth or gums together* during teething
- *Throat feels rough, narrow, hot. Tonsils swollen*
- *Shooting pain into the ears on swallowing.* Cannot swallow anything hot
- Throat feels very hot, pain at root of tongue extending to ear
- Urine scanty and suppressed with pain in kidney region
- *Breast hard swollen and very sensitives*
- Disposition to boils

Silica 30
4 pills three times daily for one month

Symptoms
- Mainly useful for the treatment of chronic rheumatism and arthritis

- Bruised pain in whole body, in the morning before walking, better on rising
- Bruised pain in all muscles of the body
- Loss of power in legs
- Heaviness and weariness of lower limbs
- Pain in knee, as if tightly bound
- Calves tense and contracted
- Sole sores
- Soreness in feet
- Pain in great toes so that he can scarcely step on them
- Cramps in calves and soles
- *Icy cold and sweaty feet*
- Pain with weakness of joints, worse upper extremities or the ankle joint
- Biting pain in the hip extending to knee with tendency of bone pain and suppuration
- Tearing in the joint when sitting
- Cramp-like pain in the thumb joints
- Paralytic weakness of forearm
- Tremulous hands when using them

Symptoms *Worse*
- In morning
- From washing
- From cold
- On uncovering
- Lying down
- Drafts of air
- At night
- Lying on left side
- Mental work
- Motion
- New moon
- Change of weather
- Getting wet

Symptoms *Better*
- Warmth (all symptoms except gastric one which are better by cold food)
- On wrapping up head
- Summer

- Sensation in tips of fingers, as if suppurating

The following symptoms generally accompany the above symptoms...
- Useful in diseases of bones, caries and necrosis
- *Suppurative processes*, ripens abscesses since it promotes suppuration
- Ailment attended with *pus formation*
- Great sensitiveness of taking cold
- *Sensitive* to all impressions and *anxious*
- Headache better by *wrapping up warmly* and *when lying on left side*
- Pain begins at back of the head, and spreads over head and settles over eyes
- *Profuse sweat of head*
- Tendency to inflammation, swelling and suppuration of glands—cervical, auxiliary, parotid, mammary. Small wounds heal with difficulty and suppurate easily
- *Pricking as if a pin in tonsil*
- Fissures and piles painful, with *spasm of sphincter of rectum*. Constipation, *stool* come down *with difficulty, when partly expelled, recedes again*
- *Night walking*—gets up while asleep
- Violent *cough* when lying down with *thick, yellow lumpy* expectoration
- White spots on nails
- *Promotes expulsion of foreign bodies* from tissues, e.g. thorn, splinters

Ruta Graveolens 30

4 pills three times daily for one month

Symptoms

- It acts upon bone, joints producing symptoms of a rheumatic nature
- For bruises that occur on bone, e.g. chin, elbow, skull
- Pain is felt on the surface of bone, particularly places where tendons are attached to the bone
- There is bruised pain all over the body, as after a fall, worse in limbs, spine and joints
- Especially in *sprains and strains* after injury when *Arnica* and *Rhus tox.* do not help
- Tendon or ligament that have been torn or wrenched
- Pain feels closer to the bone and can be associated with hard swelling where the tendon is attached to the bone
- Pain and stiffness in *wrist* and hands
- Tearing in right wrist, worse with motion; pain in left wrist as it broken
- Bursa and ganglion of wrist
- *Veins of hands swell after eating. Fingers distorted*

Symptoms *Worse*

- Lying down especially lying on painful part
- From cold
- Cold damp weather
- Rest
- Over-excretion
- Sitting or rising from a seat
- On stooping
- Beginning to move

Symptoms *Better*

- Dry warm weather
- Warmth
- Moving about

Bursitis

- Wrenching pain in shoulder joints when the arms are allowed to hang down or when resting on them
- Pain between scapulae in the afternoon
- Tension and pressure in shoulders with stiffness in morning
- *Thighs pain when stretching the limbs;* on rising from a seat, thighs and hips so weak, they are unable to support body weight so that he falls back on the seat
- Aching pain in tendo-achilles
- *Lameness and pain in ankle* with puffy swelling
- Hamstring feels shortened
- *Tendons sore;* working leaves patient weary and weak
- Pain in bones at feet and ankles. Pain in them does not permit to step heavily
- In *Tennis elbow* pain sore, bruised with lameness, worse from exercise

The following symptoms generally accompany the above symptoms . . .

- Feeling of intense lassitude, weakness and despair
- Restless, changes position frequently when lying
- All parts of body painful as if bruised
- Eyes painful with blurred vision from fine work like sewing or reading. Eyes red, hot and painful
- Difficult stool
- Prolapus ani
- Even after urination constant urging to urinate, feels bladder full
- Backache relieved by lying flat on the back

Rhus Toxicodendron 30
4 pills three times daily for one month

Symptoms

- Hot, painful swelling of joint
- Tearing and drawing pain
- *Limbs stiff, paralysed sensation*
- Tenderness about knee joint
- Trembling after exertion
- Tingling in feet
- Loss of power in forearm and fingers
- Crawling sensation in the tips of finger
- *Tearing pain in tendons, ligament and fasciae*
- Numbness after over work and exposure
- Soreness of condyles of bones
- Pains aching, sore, bruised, tearing, shooting with heaviness, lameness and stiffness
- *Sprains, strains, torn ligaments and tendinitis*

The following symptoms generally accompany the above symptoms . . .

- *Extreme restlessness* accompanies most symptoms. Cannot stay in one position, continued change of position
- Aching in bone with fever

Symptoms *Worse*

- The cold fresh air is not tolerable
- Damp weather and after rains
- From sitting and rising from sitting position or first attempt to move
- Approach of storms
- At night, especially in bed
- After overwork and exposure
- From gardening
- Checked perspiration
- Injuries after lifting and over exertion

Bursitis

- Tongue coated, except red triangular space at tip with great thirst
- Bitter taste in mouth
- Skin eruptions—red, swollen with intense itching
- Desire for milk
- Fever of typhoid character
- General or localised glandular swelling
- Trembling and palpitation of heart when siting still
- *Sensitive to open air,* putting the hand from under the bed-cover brings on cough

Symptoms *Better*
• For external heat
• Warm compress
• From warmth of bed
• Continued movement
• Change of position
• Moving attached part·
• Rubbing
• From stretching out limbs

Acid Benzoicum 30
4 pills three times daily for one month

Symptoms
- Useful in persons with *uric acid diathesis*
- It is a useful remedy in *gouty cases;* use it when Colchicum fails
- Swelling of the wrist with gout deposits
- Gouty deposits, nodes are very painful. Nodes on joints of fingers and toes
- Tearing pain in great toe

Symptoms *Worse*
• In open air
• By uncovering
• Cold air
• Change in weather
• Motion
• Wine
• Urine scanty

- *Bunion* of great toe
- Joint cracks on motion
- Tearing pain in tendons and joints with stitches
- *Pain in tendo-achilles*
- Pain and swelling in knees
- Oedema of the lower extremities
- Pain changes position suddenly, metastasise with heart pain in the cardiac region
- Rheumatism and gout alternate with heart trouble with pain in cardiac region

Symptoms *Better*
• By heat
• Profuse urination

The following symptoms generally accompany the above symptoms . . .

- *Offensive odour* of urine accompany all symptoms
- Urine is scanty, of a dark brown colour with repulsive odour; the smell exists at the time of urination and stays long afterwards
- Dribbling of urine in old men with enlarged prostate
- Renal insufficiency. Renal colic
- Rheumatism and gout alternate with heart trouble with palpitation and pain in cardiac region
- Stool offensive and liquid

Sulphur 30

4 pills twice daily for fifteen days

Symptoms

- Rheumatic and arthritic complaints due to suppression of any skin disease
- *Painful stiffness* is main symptom, with or without effusion

Bursitis

- For preventing gouty diathesis there is no better remedy than *Sulphur*
- One of the leading remedy for synoritis
- *Hot, sweaty hands*
- Trembling of hands
- Sprained pain in wrist
- Pain in left shoulder as if joint is dislocated
- Jerking in deltoid
- Drawing pain in shoulder and arms
- Swelling in fingers in morning, sticking in tips at night; of flexure surface of right middle finger
- *Stooping shoulders*, cannot walk erect
- Tearing above the nail of left ring finger, worse in the evening
- Pains seem to ascend, is worse in mid-summer heat, on clear and cloudless days
- Sweat in armpits, smelling like garlic
- Stiffness of knees and ankles
- *Burning in soles and hands at night*
- Weakness of thighs and legs

Symptoms *Worse*
- At rest
- Around 11 a.m.
- In the morning
- At night
- Warmth of bed
- When standing
- Washing and bathing
- From alcoholic stimulants
- From weather changes
- Periodically

Symptoms *Better*
- Dry, warm weather
- In open air
- Lying on right side
- From drawing up affected limbs

- Tearing extending into middle of thigh, worse on standing and on ascending stairs
- Tearing through knee extending to feet when walking and sitting
- Sprained wrenching pain in joints with cracking and stiffness, particularly in knees and shoulders
- Sudden cramp-like, painful jerking about the hip joints with stiffness
- Tension, pain in joint on walking
- Tension in hollow of knees, as if too short, on stepping
- Inclination to cramp on stretching out feet
- Rheumatic gout with itching
- Swelling and inflammation of big toe with pain

The following symptoms generally accompany the above symptoms...

- Burning everywhere in the body especially head, palm and sole
- *Dirty, filthy people,* prone to skin disease, dry and hard hair and skin
- Children—*cannot bear to be washed or bathed*
- Aversion of being washed
- *When carefully selected remedies fail to produce a favourable effect,* especially in acute disease
- Itching eruption on the skin. Scratching is followed by burning
- *Standing is worse position* for the patients, they cannot stand
- *Complaints are relapsing*—the patient seems to get almost well but the disease returns

Bursitis

- Redness of all orifices (lips, ears, eyelids, nostrils, anus, urethra etc.) as if pressed full of blood
- Discharges are offensive in character
- The discharges both of urine and faeces is painful to parts over which it passes; *parts around anus red, excoriated*. All the orifices of the body are very red
- *Milk disagrees, craves sugar,* sweets and fatty food
- *Great acidity* and sour eructations
- *Diarrhoea,* painless, *driving out of bed early in the morning*
- *Weak, empty gone feeling* and *faints about 11 a.m.*

Calcarea Phosphorica 30

4 pills three times daily for one month

Symptoms

- Shooting, tearing and aching type of rheumatic pain in all parts of body especially knees, loins and thumb
- Pain with stiffness, coldness, *numbness and crawling sensation*
- Pain become worse by any change of weather
- Buttocks, back and limbs fall asleep
- Weary when going upstairs. Cannot rise from seat. Staggering in old people when rising from a seat
- Pain in joints and bones excited or increased by every draft of cold damp air

Symptoms *Worse*

- Exposure to cold and damp weather
- Cold air
- Melting snow
- Changeable weather
- East winds
- Mental exertion
- Dinner
- After a meal, especially juicy fruits
- Motion

+ Rheumatism of cold weather, getting well in spring and returning in autumn

Symptoms *Better*
• In summer
• Warm, dry atmosphere
• Lying down
• Rest
• Passing wind

The following symptoms generally accompany the above symptom . . .

+ For anaemic persons, especially *anaemic children* who are flabby, have cold extremities and feeble digestion
+ Children—*emaciated, unable to stand, and slow in learning to walk*
+ *Feels complaints more when thinking about them*
+ *Numbness and crawling* are characteristic sensations
+ Symptoms get worse by wet cold air and every *change of weather*
+ Headache, *worse near the region of sutures*
+ Glandular enlargement—swollen tonsils. *Adenoid growths*
+ *Craving for bacon, ham, salted or smoked meat*
+ *Much flatulence.* Flatulence temporarily relieved by sour eructations
+ Pain in abdomen *at every attempt to eat*
+ Diarrhoea from juicy fruits, during dentition *with fetid flatus*
+ White discharge in females, like *white of egg*

Causticum 30

4 pills three times daily for one month

Symptoms

+ It is mainly useful in chronic rheumatic, arthritic and paralytic affections

Bursitis

- Generally indicated by tearing, drawing pains in the muscular and fibrous tissues, with deformities about the joints, especially knee and shoulder joint
- Restlessness in night with tearing pain of joints
- Pains are severe, generally remain in one joint for a long time
- Joints are stiff
- *Rheumatic tearing in limbs*
- Burning in joints
- Dull and tearing pain in hands and arm
- Rheumatism of the jaw with great stiffness
- Unsteadiness of *muscles of forearm* and hands
- Numbness, loss of sensation in hands
- Rheumatic pain of shoulders, cannot raise hand, painful stiffness between scapulae
- Pain in nape of neck as from bruises
- *Contracted tendons*
- Weak ankles, cannot walk without suffering
- Unsteady walking and easy falling

Symptoms *Worse*
- In dry cold wind
- In clear, fine weather
- Cold air
- From motion of carriage
- Expectoration
- Walking
- New moon
- After stools

Symptoms *Better*
- By warmth, especially heat of bed
- In damp, wet weather
- Open air
- Stooping low
- Emission of flatus

- *Restless legs at night.* Cannot find a position to lie still in bed for a moment at night
- Cracking and tension in knees, stiffness in hollow of knee
- Painful stiffness in the limbs through the hips, especially on rising from a seat or from a recumbent position
- Itching on the dorsum of feet

The following symptoms generally accompany the above symptoms...
- Causticum patient is sad, hopeless, dark complexioned and *intensely sympathetic*
- *Burning, rawness* and *soreness* are characteristic
- General tendency of paralytic affection
- Restlessness at night and faint-like sinking of strength. Thus weakness progresses towards paralysis
- Paralysis of single parts—vocal cards, muscles of swallowing, of tongue, eyelids, face, bladder and extremities
- Dirty white sallow skin with warts especially on the face
- Symptoms worse on right side of body
- *Coryza with hoarseness*
- *Pimples and warts* on nose
- Aversion to sweets
- Thirst for cold water but aversion to drinking
- Menses cease at night, *flow only during day*
- *Hoarseness* with pain in chest and *loss of voice*
- Cough with *raw soreness of chest*
- Expectoration scanty, must be swallowed
- Cough with *pain in hip*, worse in evening, *better with drinking cold water*

- Difficulty of voice of singers and public speakers
- *Warts* large, bleeding easily, on tips of fingers and nose
- *Retention of urine*
- Bed wetting soon after falling asleep (during first sleep)
- Involuntary urine may also dribble while coughing or sneezing or after any excitement
- Constant mental stress, effects of shock or grief, any long standing worry

Bryonia Alba 30

4 pills three times daily for one month

Symptoms

- *Joint red, hot, swollen with stitches and tearing*
- Knees stiff and painful
- Every spot is painful on pressure
- During sprain and strain, joint is painful and swollen, distended with fluid with great stiffness
- Weariness and heaviness in all limbs and stiffness
- Swollen elbow extending as far as middle of upper arm and of forearm
- Swelling sensation in joints of fingers on writing or taking hold of anything with pain
- Heaviness and weakness of legs while walking and on standing

Symptoms *Worse*

- From least motion and touch, caused by jar, by change of position, by any effort to talk, to cough, even by moving eye balls and by winking
- Hot weather after a cold spell and warmth
- Intolerance of heat
- After eating
- Exertion
- Suppressed perspiration
- 9 p.m.
- In the morning

- ✦ Stitching pain in hip joint extending to knees
- ✦ Weariness of thigh worse ascending stairs, better descending
- ✦ *Constant motion of left arm and leg*

Symptoms *Better*
• Hard pressure and rest
• Lying on painful side
• From perspiring
• Cold things, cold air, cold water
• Darkened room

The following symptoms generally accompany the above symptoms . . .

- ✦ *Dryness of all mucous membranes* like lips, mouth, throat, nose, chest, digestive tract
- ✦ *Excessive thirst.* Drinks large quantity of cold water
- ✦ Symptom develop slowly
- ✦ Patient is irritable
- ✦ Patient wants to be left alone, wants to go home even when at home
- ✦ Delirium—talks of business
- ✦ Complaints which come on *after humiliation and anger*
- ✦ Right-sided complaints
- ✦ Physical weakness
- ✦ Nausea and faintness when rising up
- ✦ Pressure in stomach after eating, as of a stone
- ✦ Bursting, splitting headache
- ✦ Breast hot and painful, hard
- ✦ Chest painful, while coughing
- ✦ Constipation, *stool hard, dry, dark, as if burnt*
- ✦ *Stitches* and stiffness in small of back

Bursitis

+ Cough, dry, spasmodic with gagging and vomiting, after eating and drinking

Kali Iodide 30

4 pills three times daily for one month

Symptoms

+ Rheumatic pain at night and in damp weather
+ *Rheumatism of knee with effusion*
+ Severe bone pains. Gnawing pain in left leg. Bones are sensitive to touch especially shin bone (leg bone)
+ Contractions of joints
+ Pain is hips causes limping when walking
+ Gout affecting every joint with an indication that hepatic region is painful on touch
+ Sensation as if small insects were crawling on the skin of lower extremities when sitting, better lying down
+ Rheumatism in *neck, back,* feet especially heels and soles worse with cold and wet

Symptoms *Worse*
• Warm clothing
• Warm room
• At night
• Damp, wet weather
• Touch
• At rest
• Lying on painful side or on back

Symptoms *Better*
• Open air (walking in open air dose not fatigue)
• Motion

The following symptoms generally accompany the above symptoms . . .

+ It acts prominently on fibrous and connective tissues, producing infiltration oedema

- *Glandular swelling*
- Emaciation and weakness
- Headache at *sides* and *root of nose*
- Profuse, *acrid, hot, watery, thin* discharge from nose
- Saliva increased, cold food and drink, especially milk, increases the suffering
- *Larynx feel raw.* Awakes choking. *Expectoration like soap-suds, greenish*
- Pimples with red tip

Mercurius Solubilis 30

4 pills two times daily for one month

Symptoms

- It is more effective in case of acute gout
- Joints sore, pale, swollen and occasional tearing pain
- Fingers flexed especially thumb with difficulty in opening
- Weakness of limbs, he can scarcely walk
- Lancinating pain in joints
- Drawing rheumatic pain in long bones particularly where the skin is thin, worse at night
- *Trembling in extremities, especially hands,* and jerking of arms
- Boring pain in periosteum of right tibia (leg bone) and drawing pain in tibia

Symptoms *Worse*
- At night
- Warmth of bed
- Warm room
- From lying on right side
- Wet, damp weather
- Extreme of temperature
- Cold air, draft of air
- Sweating
- Daylight or firelight
- Before stool
- Sitting or walking
- During exercise

Bursitis

- Swelling of feet and leg
- Cold, clammy sweat on legs at night
- Tearing pain in hips and knees, worse in open air
- Painful stiffness of wrist
- Rheumatic pain behind sternum, *cannot lie on right side*

Symptoms *Better*
• In moderate temperature
• From rest
• During the day

The following symptoms generally accompany the above symptoms...

- Complaints worse at night from change of weather, and warmth of bed. He is *sensitive to extremes of cold and heat*
- Glandular swelling with or without suppuration
- Profuse and offensive sweating with complaints; complaints worse with sweat
- Intense thirst for cold water, with moist mouth with excessive saliva, which he is constantly swallowing
- Discharges from all body increases and are offensive
- Fetid odour from mouth, metallic taste
- Body smells offensive
- Thick, moist coated tongue with imprint of teeth
- *Tremors* and trembling everywhere from least exertion
- Tension headache, *as if bandaged*
- Gums spongy and bleed easily with pain on chewing
- Dysentery *bloody, mucous stool* (more mucous than blood in stools), *with pain and tremors*
- Skin almost constantly moist with marked tendency for ulcers, boils and pus formation in general
- Lamination with swelling of hands and feet, with anaemia

Belladonna 30

4 pills three times daily for one month

Symptoms

- It is a good remedy in acute and chronic rheumatism of an inflammatory nature
- Joints swollen, red and shining
- Shooting, tearing, aching, throbbing or bruise-like pain
- *Pain comes suddenly and disappears suddenly*
- Symptoms prefer the right side
- Shifting rheumatic pains means pain changes position from one joint to another
- Patient is extremely sensitive to touch or jar
- Shooting pain along limbs
- Jerking limbs
- Involuntary limping
- Pain with redness of eyes and face
- *Cold extremities*
- Oppressive tearing pain in shoulders
- Paralytic twitching of arms with red swelling of hands and arms
- Paralytic feeling and weakness of whole left arm

Symptoms *Worse*

- In the afternoon, after 3 p.m.
- At night, especially after midnight
- Touching the affected part
- Jar
- Noise
- Draught of air
- Lying down
- Cold
- Uncovering head
- Sudden changes from warm to cold weather
- In hot weather
- Hot sun
- While looking at bright, shining object
- While drinking

- Tearing in middle joint of right index finger or in proximal joint of left middle finger
- Unsteady while walking
- Cutting stitches in outer muscles of right thigh, just above the knee, only when sitting
- Pain in thighs and legs as if caries
- When rising from bed, legs unable to carry the body weight and he sinks to the ground
- Stitches in hip joint, as if beaten

Symptoms *Better*
• Walking in open air
• When standing up after sitting
• While leaning the head against something
• Sitting erect
• Warm application (except in headache)
• Wrapping up
• In a warm room

The following symptoms generally accompany the above symptoms . . .

- Sudden and violent onset of disease which also disappears suddenly. *Pains come on suddenly and disappear suddenly*
- For inflammatory condition with heat, redness, throbbing and burning
- Complaints from cold, dry wind, especially from exposure of head to cold wind or getting head wet
- *Great remedy for children*
- Redness of toes, eyes and of inflamed part
- Oversensitive to pain worse from slight touch, (worse from pressure of cloth, bed covering) slight movement and least jar
- Right sided remedy—Symptoms occur largely on the right side
- Great thirst for cold water but *anxiety or fear of drinking*

- ✦ Throat feels constricted, difficulty in deglutition. Tonsils enlarged
- ✦ Retention of urine, *frequent and profuse urination*
- ✦ Menses too early, too profuse and very offensive and hot
- ✦ Ticking, short, dry cough, worse at night
- ✦ Glands *swollen, tender,* red. *Boils*
- ✦ Alternate redness and paleness of skin

If there is no improvement after one month then please consult a trained homoeopathic practitioner.

Acupressure

Treatment by a trained accupressurist can bring relief from bursitis pain.

Herbal Therapy

To reduce inflammation and muscle tension, and to increase blood circulation to the affected joint. Following methods are recommended:
- ✦ Mix equal parts *lobelia* (Lobelia inflata) and *cramp* (Viburnum opulus) bark to make a tincture that you can rub into your affected area to decrease the tension
- ✦ A 5 ml tincture of following herbs; 2 parts each of willow bark, cramp bark and celery seed, along with part prickly ash, should be taken three times a day
- ✦ Eating one avocado every day until the pain subsides

Juice Therapy

- ✦ Grapes, apples and lemon juice
- ✦ 1 slice ginger root, carrots, apple juice

- Broccoli, garlic clove, carrots or tomatoes, celery and ½ green pepper juice
- Orange and apple juice

Bach Flower Therapy

To reduce the inflammation of bursitis, try the Bach flower remedy known as Rescue Remedy. Rescue Remedy is a combination of five flower essences. Apply this remedy in cream form to the painful joint three or four times a day.

Diet and Nutrition

For repairing injured tendons and bursae tissue, and for making firm tissue building these dietary sources are recommended:

- Citrus fruits—lemon, orange and grapes
- Cod-liver oil
- Broccoli, green pepper
- Carrot, parley
- Spinach, asparagus and potatoes
- Ginger root and garlic
- Pineapple

Prevention

The most effective way to avoid bursitis and other strains is warming up before strenuous exercise and cooling down afterwards.

Chapter 6

Tennis Elbow

Inflammation resulting from strain of the common extensor tendon which arises from the lateral epicondyle of the humerus (upper arm bone) is called Tennis Elbow. This condition may result from repeated strenuous and jarring movement while playing sports, or from twisting movements of the forearm in screw driving and similar activities.

This is also known as *lateral epicondylitis*. Tennis elbow was first identified by doctors more than 100 years ago. Nearly half of all tennis players suffer from this disorder. While people of all ages and races can develop tennis elbow, but middle aged athletes and manual workers like carpenters and house painters, are at greatest risk. Middle age women who do piece work in the garment industry are also highly susceptible.

Due to playing computer games for long time children may also suffer from tennis elbow. Office workers who use a computer for typing intensely for long hours are also susceptible. Initially, a part of tendon and the muscle covering have minor tears. Generally, first injury heals but again the chances of injury in this area are more. Repeated injury causes bleeding in this area and there is formation of rough, granulated tissue and calcium deposits within the surrounding area. Pressure develops due to inflammation which can cut off the blood flow and irritate the radial nerve, one of the major nerve controlling muscles in the arm and hand. Tendons do not receive the required amount of oxygen and blood supply as compared to muscles, so they heal more slowly. Tendons attach muscles to bones. (*See figure 6.1*).

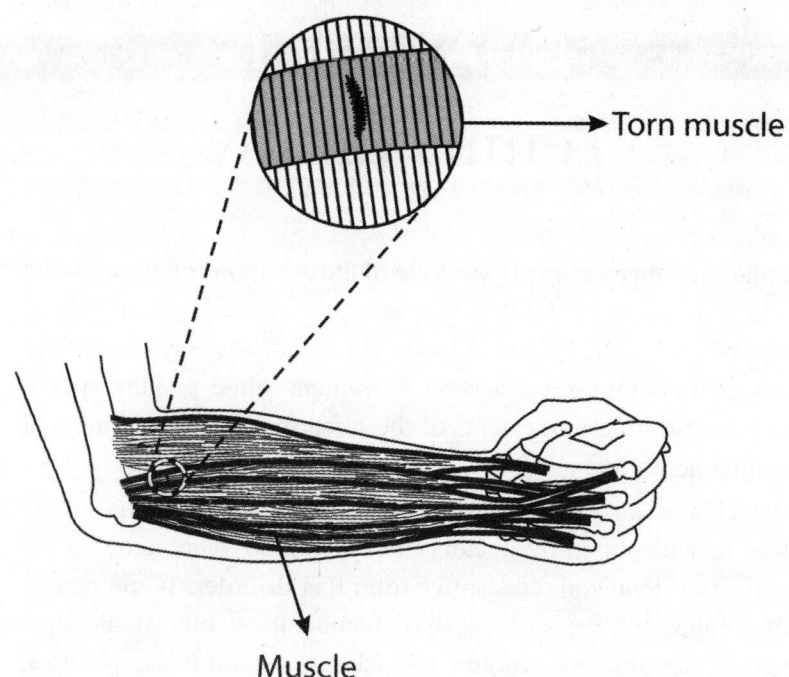

Fig. 6.1 *Excessive Pressure and Stress can Cause the Muscle to Tear*

Tennis Elbow

Causes

- *Tennis players*—they have great deal of stress on relatively delicate tendons located on the outside of elbow and on the muscle which helps control the wrist
- Making aggressive twist with a screwdriver or other implements. House painters, carpenters
- Lifting heavy objects with your elbow locked and your arm extended
- People over 30 are more likely to suffer because younger people have more supple joints
- Those who work a lot with their hands

Symptoms

- Recurring pain on the outside of the upper part of forearm just below the bend of the elbow. Sometimes pain radiates downwards toward the wrist
- Pain caused by bending the arm
- Pain caused by lifting the arm
- Pain caused by grasping even light object such as a tea cup
- Swelling is almost never a symptom of tennis elbow
- Difficulty extending the forearm fully
- Some cases of tennis elbow can last for years though the inflammation usually subsides in 6 to 12 weeks

Consult a Doctor if

- The pain persists for more than a few days at the elbow joint and just below the bend of elbow

✦ Elbow joint begins to swell, so you may think of other conditions such as arthritis, gout because tennis elbow rarely causes swelling

Treatment and Management

Most basic things to relieve the pain in tennis elbow are: *Rest* the arm until the pain disappears, *massage* to relieve stress and tension in the muscles and *exercise* to strengthen the area to prevent recurrence. Before starting any activity be sure to warm up your arm for at least 5 to 10 minutes with gentle stretching and movement.

Homoeopathy

✦ Massage the arm with *Rhus tox.* ointment to relieve pain

The following remedies are generally indicated in tennis elbow treatment:

Rhus Toxicodendron 30

4 pills three times daily for one month

Symptoms

✦ Hot, painful swelling of joint
✦ Tearing and drawing pain
✦ *Limbs stiff, paralysed sensation*
✦ Tenderness about knee joint
✦ Trembling after exertion
✦ Tingling in feet

Symptoms *Worse*
- The cold fresh air is not tolerable
- Damp weather and after rains
- From sitting and rising from sitting position or first attempt to move
- Approach of storms
- At night, especially in bed
- After overwork and exposure
- From gardening
- Checked perspiration
- Injuries after lifting and over exertion

Tennis Elbow

- Loss of power in forearm and fingers
- Crawling sensation in the tips of fingers
- *Tearing pain in tendons, ligament and fasciae*
- Numbness after over work and exposure
- Soreness of condyles of bones
- Pains aching, sore, bruised, tearing, shooting with heaviness, lameness and stiffness
- *Sprains, strains, torn ligaments and tendinitis*

Symptoms *Better*
• For external heat
• Warm compress
• From warmth of bed
• Continued movement
• Change of position
• Moving affected part
• Rubbing
• From stretching out limbs

The following symptoms generally accompany the above symptoms . . .

- *Extreme restlessness* accompanies most symptoms. Cannot stay in one position, continuous change of position
- Aching in bone with fever
- Tongue coated, except red triangular space at tip with great thirst
- Bitter taste in mouth
- Skin eruptions—red, swollen with intense itching
- Desire for milk
- Fever of typhoid character
- General or localised glandular swelling
- Trembling and palpitation of heart when siting still
- Sensitive to open air, putting the hand from under the bed-cover brings on cough

Ruta Graveolens 30

4 pills three times daily for one month

Symptoms

- It acts upon bone, joints producing symptoms of a rheumatic nature
- For bruises that occurs on bone, e.g. chin, elbow, skull
- Pain is felt on surface of bone, particularly places where tendons are attached to the bone
- There is bruised pain all over the body, as after a fall, worse in limbs, spine and joints
- Especially in *sprains and strains* after injury when *Arnica* and *Rhus tox.* do not help
- Tendon or ligament that have been torn or wrenched
- Pain feels closer to the bone and can be associated with hard swelling where the tendon is attached to the bone
- Pain and stiffness in *wrist* and hands
- Tearing in right wrist, worse with motion; pain in left wrist as if broken
- Bursa and ganglion of wrist
- *Veins of hands swell after eating. Fingers distorted*

Symptoms *Worse*

- Lying down especially lying on painful part
- From cold
- Cold damp weather
- Rest
- Over-excretion
- Sitting or rising from a seat
- On stooping
- Beginning to move

Symptoms *Better*

- Dry warm weather
- Warmth
- Moving about

- Wrenching pain in shoulder joints when the arms are allowed to hang down or when resting on them
- Pain between scapulae in the afternoon
- Tension and pressure in shoulders with stiffness in the morning
- *Thighs pain when stretching the limbs;* on rising from seat, thighs and hips are weak, they are unable to support body weight so that the patient falls back on the seat
- Aching pain in tendo-achilles
- *Lameness and pain in ankle* with puffy swelling
- Hamstring feels shortened
- *Tendons sore;* working leaves patient weary and weak
- Pain in bones at feet and ankles. Pain in them does not permit to step heavily
- In *Tennis elbow* pain sore, bruised with lameness, worse from exercise

The following symptoms generally accompany the above symptoms . . .

- Feeling of intense lassitude, weakness and despair
- Restless, changes position frequently when lying
- All parts of body painful as if bruised
- Eyes painful with blurred vision from fine work like sewing or reading. Eyes red, hot and painful
- Difficult stool
- Prolapus ani
- Even after urination constant urging to urinate, feels bladder full
- Backache relieved by lying flat on the back

Magnesia Phosphorica 30

4 pills three times daily for one month

Symptoms
- Neuralgic pain and cramping of muscles
- In sprain and strain sharp, stabbing, shooting pain
- Pain generally sharp, cutting, piercing, knife like, stabbing, shooting, stitching, lightening like
- Involuntary shaking of hands
- Cramps in calves
- Writer's and player's cramp
- Weakness in arms and legs
- Finger tips numb and stiff
- General muscular weakness

Symptoms *Worse*
• On the right side
• Touch
• At night
• Cold bathing or washing
• Being uncovered
• Walking in fresh air

Symptoms *Better*
• Warmth and heat
• Bending double
• Pressure
• Friction

The following symptoms generally accompany the above symptoms . . .

- Suitable for lean thin emaciated persons who are forgetful, easily tired, drowsy, averse to mental effort
- Main remedy for *spasmodic pain; pain generally sudden and severe*
- Painful ailment relieved by the *application of heat*
- Pain shifts rapidly and usually affects right side of the body
- Craving for sugar, averse to coffee
- May have thirst for cold drinks
- *Menstrual cramping* better after the flow begins

- Indicated for *all forms of cramp,* spasmodic and neuralgic pains in head, face, teeth, abdomen or stomach
- A fine remedy for the tummy pains of babies
- Flatulent colic, forcing the patient to bend double, accompanied with belching of gas, which gives no relief. Bloated abdomen, must loosen cloth, walk about and constantly pass flatus
- Spasmodic cough, whooping cough
- Angia pectoris
- In fever, chills run up and down the back with shivering
- Great dread of cold air, *of uncovering,* of touching affected part, of cold bathing or walking, of moving

Causticum 30
4 pills three times daily for one month

Symptoms
- It is mainly useful in chronic rheumatic, arthritic and paralytic affections
- Generally indicated by tearing, drawing pains in the muscular and fibrous tissues, with deformities about the joints, especially knee and shoulder joint
- Restlessness in night with tearing pain of joints
- Pains are severe, generally remain in one joint for a long time
- Joints are stiff

Symptoms *Worse*
• In dry cold wind
• In clear, fine weather
• Cold air
• From motion of carriage
• Expectoration
• Walking
• New moon
• After stools

- *Rheumatic tearing in limbs*
- Burning in joints
- Dull and tearing pain in hands and arm
- Rheumatism of the jaw with great stiffness
- Unsteadiness of *muscles of forearm* and hands
- Numbness, loss of sensation in hands
- Rheumatic pain of shoulders, cannot raise hand, painful stiffness between scapulae
- Pain in nape of neck as from bruises
- *Contracted tendons*
- Weak ankles, cannot walk without suffering
- Unsteady walking and easy falling
- *Restless legs at night.* Cannot find a position to lie still in bed for a moment at night
- Cracking and tension in knees, stiffness in hollow of knee
- Painful stiffness in the limbs through the hips, especially on rising from a seat or from a recumbent position
- Itching on the dorsum of feet

Symptoms *Better*
• By warmth, especially heat of bed
• In damp, wet weather
• Open air
• Stooping low
• Emission of flatus

The following symptoms generally accompany the above symptoms . . .

- Causticum patient is sad, hopeless, dark complexioned and *intensely sympathetic*
- *Burning, rawness* and *soreness* are characteristic
- General tendency of paralytic affection

- Restlessness at night and faint-like sinking of strength. Thus weakness progresses towards paralysis
- Paralysis of single parts—vocal cards, muscles of swallowing, of tongue, eyelids, face, bladder and extremities
- Dirty white sallow skin with warts especially on the face
- Symptoms worse on right side of body
- *Coryza with hoarseness*
- *Pimples and warts* on nose
- Aversion to sweets
- Thirst for cold water but aversion to drinking
- Menses cease at night, *flow only during day*
- *Hoarseness* with pain in chest and *loss of voice*
- Cough with *raw soreness of chest*
- Expectoration scanty, must be swallowed
- Cough with *pain in hip*, worse in evening, *better with drinking cold water*
- Difficulty of voice of singers and public speakers
- *Warts* large, bleeding easily, on tips of fingers and nose
- *Retention of urine*
- Bed wetting soon after falling sleep (during first sleep)
- Involuntary urine may also double while coughing or sneezing or after any excitement
- Constant mental stress, effects of shock or grief any long standing worry

Pulsatilla 30

4 pills three times daily for one month

Symptoms

- Drawing, tearing pains in joints with swelling and redness, especially hips, knees, elbows and small joints of hand and feet
- The *pains shift* rapidly *from one part to another*
- Can hardly give symptoms and starts crying
- Rheumatic pains are so severe that the patient is compelled to move slowly, as easy motion relieves pain
- Drawing, tensive pain in thighs and legs with restlessness and *chilliness*
- *Pain in limbs*, tensive pain, *letting up with a snap*
- Pain appears in a part, increases to a climax and then disappears suddenly from the part
- Pain in limbs in the morning in bed on waking with stiffness
- Hip-joint painful
- Knees swollen, with tearing, drawing pains
- Boring pain in heels like pricking of nails towards evening, *suffering worse from letting the affected limb hang down*
- Feet red, inflamed and swollen
- Numbness around elbow

Symptoms *Worse*

- From heat
- Rich fat food
- After eating
- In warm close room
- Evening
- At twilight
- Lying on left or on painless side
- When allowing feet to hand down
- At beginning to move
- On being seated or flexing (back)

- Tearing in the shoulder joint obliging him to bend arms, extends intermittently to wrists and fingers
- Legs feel heavy and weary
- Nervousness, intensely felt about the ankles

Symptoms *Better*
- Cool open air
- Slow motion
- Cold application
- Cold food and drink
- Lying on the painful side
- Pressure or tying up tightly especially in the head
- Rest

The following symptoms generally accompany the above symptoms . . .

- Very often indicated in the later, established stage of illness
- It is pre-eminently a female remedy, especially for mild gentle, sad, crying, readily *weeps when talking, changeable,* contradictory
- Feels better by consolation
- The patient is chilly but she *feels better in open air and seeks the open air*
- Dry mouth but absence of thirst with nearly all complaints
- *Secretion* from all mucous membranes are *thick, bland and yellowish-green*
- *Symptoms ever changing*—no two stools, no two attacks alike; very well one hour, very miserable the next
- Pains *rapidly shifting* from one part to another
- Eyes inflamed and agglutinated, styes
- Cracks in middle of lower lips. *Yellow or white tongue,* covered with a tenacious mucous
- Desire for rich and fatty food, which leads to indigestion

- Dry cough in the evening and at night, must sit up in bed to get relief and loose cough in the morning. Pressure upon the chest and soreness
- Menses too late, scanty or suppressed
- Useful remedy to begin the treatment in a chronic case

Arnica Montana 30

4 pills three times daily for one month

Symptoms

- Rheumatism of muscular and tendinous tissue, especially of hip, back and shoulders
- It is suited to cases when any injury, however remote, seems to have caused the present trouble. *After traumatic injury*
- A muscular tonic
- Limbs and body aches as if beaten; joints as if sprained
- *Sore, lame and brushed feeling*
- Sharp, shooting, paralytic or sprained pains which quickly change place
- *Gouty affections.* Great fear at being touched or approached
- Sore, tender, red swelling of the joints in gout, particularly of knee joint
- Gout with arthritic pains in the feet and the big toe as if sprained

Symptoms *Worse*
• Least touch
• Motion
• Rest
• Wine
• Damp cold
• Evening
• From speaking
• Blowing nose
• Almost any noise
• Lying on injured part
• From over excretion
• Alcohol
• Old age

Tennis Elbow

- In arthritis especially hip joint is affected
- Rheumatism begins low down and works up
- Cannot walk erect, on account of bruised pain in pelvic region
- Paralytic pains in all joints during motion
- Knee bends suddenly when walking, stitches when touched
- Twitching pain from left shoulder joint to the middle finger
- Pain in back and limbs, as if bruised
- Deathly coldness of forearms
- Everything on which the patient lies seems too hard
- Soreness after over-exertion
- Cracking in the right wrist when the hand is moved, as if dislocated
- During *Sprains* and *Strains* ligaments torn with swelling which is most prominent. Bruising and inflammation of the soft tissue around the joint
- When muscles or soft tissues are black and blue

Symptoms *Better*
• Lying down
• Lying with head low
• Warmth
• Rubbing and wrapping up warmly
• Long walk in cold weather
• Out stretched
• From changing position

Following symptoms generally accompany the above symptoms . . .

- Produces conditions similar to those resulting from injuries, falls, blows, contusions

- Especially suited to cases when any injury occurs; *after any traumatic injuries*
- Remote effects of injuries even though received years ago
- Whole body feels *sore and bruised, lame* and does not want to be approached, touched or jarred
- It *promotes healing,* reduces swelling, prevents pus formation
- It is very effective in bleeding of any kind
- *Head hot with cold body*
- Fetid breath
- Diarrhoea offensive and bloody
- *Violent spasmodic cough with facial herpes*
- Skin *black and blue.* Multiple small boils very painful. Acne characterised by *symmetry in distribution*
- *Aids recovery after an operation*

Silica 30
4 pills three times daily for one month

Symptoms
- Mainly useful for the treatment of chronic rheumatism and arthritis
- Bruised pain in whole body, in the morning before walking, better rising
- Bruised pain in all muscles of body
- Loss of power in legs
- Heaviness and weariness of lower limbs
- Pain in knee, as if tightly bound
- Calves tense and contracted
- Sole sores

- Soreness in feet
- Pain in great toes so that the patient can scarcely step on them
- Cramps in calves and soles
- *Icy cold and sweaty feet*
- Pain with weakness of joints, worse upper extremities or the ankle joint
- Biting pain in the hip extending to knee with tendency of bone pain and suppuration
- Tearing in the joint when sitting
- Cramp-like pain in the thumb joints
- Paralytic weakness of forearm
- Tremulous hands when using them
- Sensation in tips of fingers, as if suppurating

The following symptoms generally accompany the above symptoms . . .

- Useful in diseases of bones, caries and necrosis
- *Suppurative processes*, ripens abscesses since it promotes suppuration
- Ailment attended with *pus formation*

Symptoms *Worse*
- In morning
- From washing
- From cold
- On uncovering
- Lying down
- Drafts of air
- At night
- Lying on left side
- Mental work
- Motion
- New moon
- Change of weather
- Getting wet

Symptoms *Better*
- Warmth (all symptoms except gastric one which are better by cold food)
- On wrapping up the head
- Summer

- Great sensitiveness of taking cold
- *Sensitive* to all impressions and *anxious*
- Headache better by *wrapping up warmly* and *when lying on left side*
- Pain begins at back of head, and spreads all over head and settles over eyes
- *Profuse sweat of head*
- Tendency to inflammation, swelling and suppuration of glands—cervical, auxiliary, parotid, mamary. Small wounds heal with difficulty and suppurate easily
- *Pricking as if a pin in tonsil*
- Fissures and piles painful, with *spasm of sphincter of rectum*. Constipation, *stool* come down *with difficulty, when partly expelled, recedes again*
- *Night walking*—gets up while asleep
- Violent *cough* when lying down with *thick, yellow lumpy* expectoration
- White spots on nails
- *Promotes expulsion of foreign bodies* from tissues, e.g. thorn, splinters.

Following an analysis of overall situation you can take remedies that may relieve pain and other symptoms. If there is no improvement after taking remedies then please consult a trained homoeopathic practitioner.

Acupressure

Deep thumb pressure on Large Instine II point, located inside the elbow, may relieve pain.

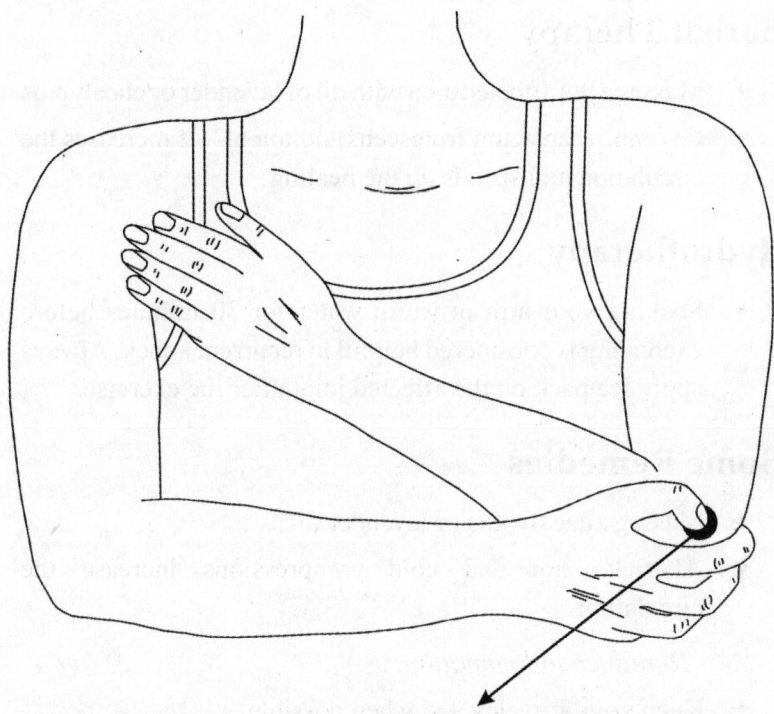

Large Intestine II

Fig. 6.2 *Tennis Elbow*

Physiotherapy

They commonly use diathermy (a form of electrical stimulation), ultrasound rays, and massage to treat tennis elbow.

Electric current and sound improves circulation and drainage, which makes it easier to stretch and massage the affected area.

Sometimes, physiotherapist prescribes a splint or band to take stress off the affected area during relevant activities. Wearing the splint for a longer period can hamper the blood flow of the affected area and slow down the recovery.

Herbal Therapy

- Massage the affected area with oil of lavender or eucalyptus
- Cayenne (capsicum frutescens) ointment—It increases the circulation and speeds up the healing

Hydrotherapy

- Soaking your arm in warm water for 30 minutes before exercising is considered helpful in recurrent attack. Always apply ice pack on the affected joint after the exercise.

Home Remedies

- Massage eucalyptus or lavender oil
- Alternate hot and cold compressions increase the circulation

To reduce inflammation:

- Keep your arm elevated when possible
- Ask someone to massage the most painful part of your elbow with the convex side of a spoon aggressively. This causes lots of pain at first but eventually dulls the nerve ending and reduces the inflammation

Prevention

Preventing a tennis elbow

If you work a lot with your hands, you may wish to take these precautionary measures:

- Lift objects with your palm facing your body
- Try strengthening exercises with hand weights. With your elbow locked and your palm down, repeatedly bend your wrist. Stop if you feel any pain
- Before a stressful activity stretch relevant muscles by grasping the top part of your fingers and gently but firmly pulling them back toward your body with your arm fully extended and palm facing outward

Preventing relapse

- Discontinue the activities that cause stress on your elbow joint. Warm up for 10 minute before any activity involving your arm and apply ice to it afterwards. Take frequent breaks
- Tie splint or band around your forearm during relevant activities like lifting objects such as heavy books. Be aware that prolong use of band can cut off circulation

Chapter 7

Carpal Tunnel Syndrome

Carpal tunnel syndrome is defined as soreness, tenderness, and weakness in thumbs and first three fingers caused by pressure on the median nerve at the point where it goes though the carpal tunnel of the wrist.

This tunnel lies on the palm side of the wrist and is formed by the arch of the wrist bones behind and a strong band of fibrous tissue in front. Blood vessels and the tendons of the muscles that flex the fingers also pass through the carpal tunnel. Pressure in the tunnel increases if the tendons thicken or if its cavity is narrowed.

Numbness, tingling and burning sensations are its characteristic symptoms. Sometimes the wrist, elbow and other joints are also affected. This is due to repetitive, unrelieved motion of the hands such as sitting at a computer keyboard and typing all the time, especially by officer workers or carpenters. These symptoms are experienced generally at night, after the regular workday or when you are ready to go to sleep. There is a feeling of clumsiness in carrying out fine movements.

If treatment is not given on time, the symptoms progress to persistent pain and aching in the other areas such as hands and arms, and eventually lead to the inability to grip things firmly and to use your hands in a normal way.

If the same symptoms are present in your feet, ankle and lower legs the condition is known as *tarsal tunnel syndrome*. Other causes of carpal tunnel syndrome include injury to the wrist, inflammation, rheumatoid arthritis, swellings, some systemic diseases and nutrient deficiency. Carpal tunnel syndrome is most common in the middle age and tends to affect women more than men, especially if the woman are overweight, pregnant or after menopause. It is important to remove the cause of this disease if at all possible. For some, this may require a change of job if the current job involves repetitive use of hands. Failure to do so results in permanent, irreversible damage to the nerve and muscles of the hands and wrist. Carpal tunnel syndrome is also known as repetitive stress injury. (*See figures 7.1 and 7.2*).

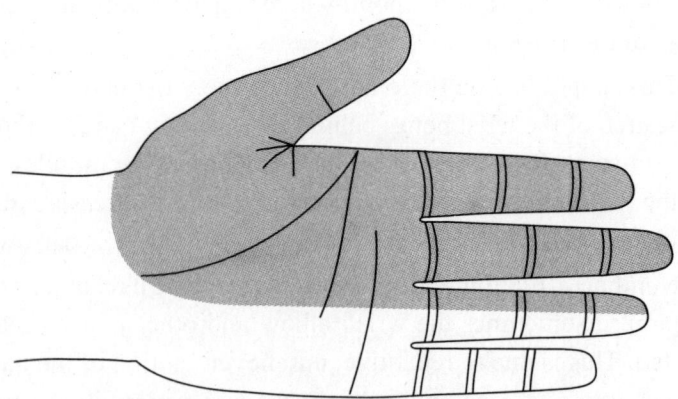

Fig. 7.1 *Showing Affected Area When Median Nerve is Stressed or Pinched*

Carpel Tunnel Syndrome

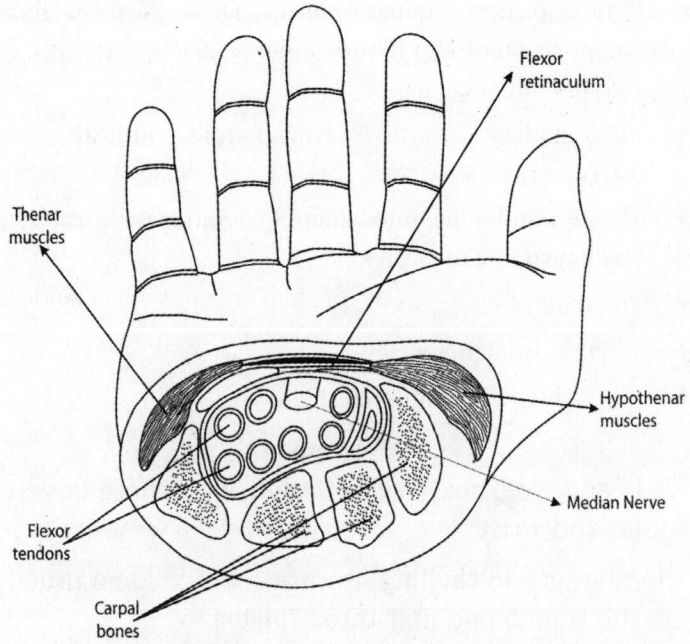

Fig. 7.2 *The Carpal Tunnel*

Causes

+ Stressful position of hand, arm and neck, such as working at a desk, long-distance driving or waiting on tables
+ Working for long periods with steady hand movement, from musicians to meat cutters. Their work demands repeated grasping, turning, and twisting or involving repetitive vibration, as in hammering nails or operating a power tool
+ Sports that cause repetitive stress injuries include—rowing, golf, tennis, downhill skiing, archery, competitive shooting, and rock climbing etc. These activities stress the hand and wrist joint

- Injuries or post traumatic causes: These cause swelling or compression of soft tissue on nerves such as sprains, after a colles fracture
- Inflammatory causes: Rheumatoid arthritis, wrist osteoarthritis, leukemia
- Thyroid problems, myxoedema, acromegaly, diabetes and other systemic disorders
- Pregnancy
- Vitamin B6 deficiency
- Idiopathic—the commonest cause

Symptoms

- Pain and weakness in the thumb, first three fingers, palm and wrist
- Numbness and tingling sensation in the hand usually in the thumb and first three fingers.
- Pain often worse at night or before sleep, usually after exertion at work place
- Shooting pain in the wrist, forearm and sometimes extending to the shoulder, neck and chest
- Feeling of clumsiness in carrying out fine movements
- Difficulty in clenching the fist or grasping small objects
- Sometimes—dry skin and deterioration of fingernails

Consult a Doctor if

- Your hands or fingers feel painful, numb and stiff, the joints have become swollen; you may be suffering from a form of arthritis

- After a fall or other accident, you feel pain in your wrist, hand or fingers. You may have a broken bone
- Pain is more intense at night; you may have diabetes
- The skin on your hands and fingers becomes white and then bright red, especially in cold weather

Lab Investigations

- Doctor will check for swelling, inflammation, weakness, limited range of movement and poor reflexes in the hands and arm
- Tinel's sign test—tapping the front of wrist causes numbness in the forearm of a carpal tunnel syndrome patient
- Wrist flexion test—also known as reverse prayer test. Holding the hands together back to back, with finger nails touching, induces tingling in a patient
- When a blood pressure cuff is inflated above systolic pressure on the forearm, a pain or numbness is induced due to compression. This procedure also confirms the condition of a carpal tunnel syndrome patient
- X-ray and MRI (Magnetic Resonance Imaging)
- Nerve Conducting Velocity (NCV) studies show delayed or absent conduction of impulses in the median nerve across the wrist
- Electromyograph (EMG)

Treatment and Management

- It is important for people with carpal tunnel syndrome to avoid activities that involve forceful wrist-bending. Patient

- is advised rest, cool baths or cold compression, wearing wrist splint especially during sleep
- In some cases, the doctor may recommend that you stop typing or doing hand/finger work until the symptoms subside
- You can use a wrist support in front of computer keyboard
- Take frequent breaks to relieve stress

Homoeopathy

The following remedies are usually indicated in carpal tunnel syndrome. Following an analysis of overall situation you can take remedies that may relieve the pain and other symptoms.

Pulsatilla 30

4 pills three times daily for one month

Symptoms

- Drawing, tearing pains in joints with swelling and redness, especially hips, knees, elbows and small joints of hand and feet
- The *pains shift* rapidly *from one part to another*
- Can hardly give symptoms and starts crying
- Rheumatic pains are so severe that the patient is compelled to move slowly, as easy motion relieves pain
- Drawing, tensive pain in thighs and legs with restlessness and *chilliness*

Symptoms *Worse*
- From heat
- Rich fat food
- After eating
- In warm close room
- Evening
- At twilight
- Lying on left or on painless side
- When allowing feet to hang down
- When beginning to move
- On being seated or flexing (back)

Carpel Tunnel Syndrome

- *Pain in limbs*, tensive pain, *letting up with a snap*
- Pain appears in a part, increases to a climax and then disappears suddenly from the part
- Pain in limbs in the morning in bed on waking with stiffness
- Hip-joint painful
- Knees swollen, with tearing, drawing pains
- Boring pain in heels like pricking of nails towards evening, *suffering worse from letting the affected limb hang down*
- Feet red inflamed and swollen
- Numbness around elbow
- Tearing in the shoulder joint obliging him to bend arms, extends intermittently to wrists and fingers
- Legs feel heavy and weary
- Nervousness, intensely felt about the ankles

Symptoms *Better*
• Cool open air
• Slow motion
• Cold application
• Cold food and drink
• Lying on painful side
• Pressure or tying up tightly especially in head
• Rest

The following symptoms generally accompany the above symptoms . . .

- Very often indicated in the later, established stage of illness
- It is pre-eminently a female remedy, especially for mild, gentle, sad, crying, readily *weeps when talking, changeable,* contradictory
- Feels better by consolation
- The patient is chilly but she *feels better in open air and seeks the open air*

- ✦ Dry mouth but absence of thirst with nearly all complaints. *Secretion* from all mucous membranes are *thick, bland and yellowish-green*
- ✦ *Symptoms ever changing*—no two stools, no two attacks alike; very well one hour, very miserable the next
- ✦ Pains *rapidly shifting* from one part to another
- ✦ Eyes inflamed and agglutinated, styes
- ✦ Cracks in middle of lower lips. *Yellow or white tongue*, covered with a tenacious mucous
- ✦ Desire for rich and fatty food, which leads to indigestion
- ✦ Dry cough in the evening and at night, must sit up in bed to get relief and loose cough in the morning. Pressure upon the chest and soreness
- ✦ Menses too late, scanty or suppressed
- ✦ Useful remedy to begin the treatment in a chronic case

Rhus Toxicodendron 30

4 pills three times daily for one month

Symptoms

- ✦ Hot, painful swelling of joint
- ✦ Tearing and drawing pain
- ✦ *Limbs stiff, paralysed sensation*
- ✦ Tenderness about knee joint
- ✦ Trembling after exertion
- ✦ Tingling in feet

Symptoms *Worse*

- The cold fresh air is not tolerable
- Damp weather and after rains
- From sitting and rising from sitting position or first attempt to move
- Approach of storms
- At night, especially in bed
- After overwork and exposure
- From gardening
- Checked perspiration
- Injuries after lifting and over exertion

Carpel Tunnel Syndrome

- Loss of power in forearm and fingers
- Crawling sensation in the tips of fingers
- *Tearing pain in tendons, ligament and fasciae*
- Numbness after over work and exposure
- Soreness of condyles of bones
- Pains aching, sore, bruised, tearing, shooting with heaviness, lameness and stiffness
- *Sprains, strains, torn ligaments and tendinitis*

Symptoms *Better*
• From external heat
• Warm compresses
• From warmth of bed
• Continued movement
• Change of position
• Moving affected part
• Rubbing
• From stretching out limbs

The following symptoms generally accompany the above symptoms...

- *Extreme restlessness* accompanies most symptoms. Cannot stay in one position, continued change of position
- Aching in bone with fever
- Tongue coated, except red triangular space at tip with great thirst
- Bitter taste in mouth
- Skin eruptions—red, swollen with intense itching
- Desire for milk
- Fever of typhoid character
- General or localised glandular swelling
- Trembling and palpitation of heart when siting still
- *Sensitive to open air,* putting the hand from under the bedcover brings on cough

Ruta Graveolens 30

4 pills three times daily for one month

Symptoms

+ It acts upon bone, joints producing symptoms of a rheumatic nature
+ For bruises that occurs on bone, e.g. chin, elbow, skull
+ Pain is felt on the surface of bone, particularly in places where tendons are attached to the bone
+ There is bruised pain all over the body, as after a fall, worse in limbs, spine and joints
+ Especially in *sprains and strains* after injury when *Arnica* and *Rhus tox.* do not help
+ Tendon or ligament that have been torn or wrenched
+ Pain feels closer to the bone and can be associated with hard swelling where the tendon is attached to the bone
+ Pain and stiffness in *wrist* and hands
+ Tearing in right wrist, worse with motion; pain in left wrist as it broken
+ Bursa and ganglion in wrist

Symptoms *Worse*

- Lying down especially lying on the painful part
- From cold
- Cold damp weather
- Rest
- Over-excretion
- Sitting or rising from a seat
- On stooping
- Beginning to move

Symptoms *Better*

- Dry warm weather
- Warmth
- Moving about

- *Veins of hands swell after eating. Fingers distorted*
- Wrenching pain in shoulder joints when the arms are allowed to hang down or when resting on them
- Pain between scapulae in the afternoon
- Tension and pressure in shoulders with stiffness in the morning
- *Thighs pain when stretching the limbs;* on rising from a seat, thighs and hips so weak, they are unable to support body weight so that he falls back on the seat
- Aching pain in tendo-achilles
- *Lameness and pain in ankle* with puffy swelling
- Hamstring feel shortened
- *Tendons sore;* working leaves patient weary and weak
- Pain in bones at feet and ankles. Pain in them does not permit to step heavily
- In *Tennis elbow* pain sore, bruised with lameness, worse from exercise

The following symptoms generally accompany the above symptoms...

- Feeling of intense lassitude, weakness and despair
- Restless, changes position frequently when lying
- All parts of body painful as if bruised
- Eyes painful with blurred vision from fine work like sewing or reading. Eyes red, hot and painful
- Difficult stool
- Prolapus ani
- Even after urination constant urging to urinate, feels bladder full
- Backache relieved by lying flat on the back

Arnica Montana 30

4 pills three times daily for one month

Symptoms

- Rheumatism of muscular and tendinous tissue, especially of hip, back and shoulders
- It is suited to cases when any injury, however remote, seems to have caused the present trouble. *After traumatic injury*
- A muscular tonic
- Limbs and body aches as if beaten; joints as if sprained
- *Sore, lame and bruised feeling*
- Sharp, shooting, paralytic or sprained pains which quickly change place
- *Gouty affections.* Great fear at being touched or approached
- Sore, tender, red swelling of the joints in gout, particularly of knee joint
- Gout with arthritic pains in the feet and the big toe as if sprained
- In arthritis, especially the hip joint is affected
- Rheumatism begins low down and works up
- Cannot walk erect, on account of bruised pain in pelvic region
- Paralytic pains in all joints during motion
- Knee bends suddenly when walking, stitches when touched

Symptoms *Worse*
• By least touch
• Motion
• Rest
• Wine
• Damp cold
• In the evening
• From speaking
• Blowing nose
• Almost any noise
• Lying on injured part
• From over-exertion
• Alcohol
• Old age

- Twitching pain from left shoulder joint to middle finger
- Pain in back and limbs, as if bruised
- Deathly coldness of forearms
- Everything on which he lies seems too hard
- Soreness after over-exertion
- Cracking in the right wrist when the hand is moved, as if it is dislocated
- During *Sprains* and *Strains* ligaments torn with swelling which is most prominent. Bruising and inflammation of the soft tissue around the joint
- When muscles or soft tissues are black and blue

Symptoms *Better*
• Lying down
• Lying with head low
• Warmth
• Rubbing and wrapping up warmly
• Long walk in cold weather
• Out stretched
• Changing position

Following symptoms generally accompany the above symptoms . . .

- Produces conditions similar to those resulting from injuries, falls, blows, contusions
- Especially suited to cases when any injury occurs; *after any traumatic injuries*
- Remote effects of injuries even though received years ago
- Whole body feels *sore and bruised, lame* and does not want to be approached, touched or jarred
- It *promotes healing,* reduces swelling, prevents pus formation
- It is very effective in bleeding of any kind
- *Head hot with cold body*

- ✦ Fetid breath
- ✦ Diarrhoea offensive and bloody
- ✦ *Violent spasmodic cough with facial herpes*
- ✦ Skin *black and blue*. Multiple small boils very painful. Acne characterised by *symmetry in distribution*
- ✦ *Aids recovery after an operation*

Calcarea Carbonica 30

4 pills three times daily for one month

Symptoms

- ✦ It is a useful remedy for rheumatoid arthritis, chronic and acute muscular rheumatism, gouty nodosities
- ✦ Rheumatic pains, after getting wet
- ✦ Sharp sticking pain, as if parts were sprained
- ✦ *Cold, damp feet,* feels as if damp stockings were worn
- ✦ Pains are shooting, cutting or tearing, sometimes confined to small spots
- ✦ Pains are associated with cramps, contraction, stiffness and weakness all over the body
- ✦ Cold knees
- ✦ Cramp in calves
- ✦ Sour foot sweat

Symptoms *Worse*
- From exertion, mental or physical
- Ascending
- Cold in every form
- Washing, moist air, wet weather
- During full moon
- Standing
- After eating
- In the evening, after midnight

- Swelling of joints, especially knee
- Inflammation of hip joints which is painfully sore
- Burning of soles of feet which feel cold and dead at night
- Weakness in the muscles of thigh in the morning, on beginning to walk, with stiffness, *worse while ascending stairs or any height*
- Pain in calves on stepping, on touch and on bending foot
- *Soles of feet raw*
- Ankles weary, feels as if dislocated
- Tearing in muscles
- Rheumatoid arthritis of finger joints with swelling and arthritic nodosities on hand and finger joints
- Pain in upper arm, as if beaten
- Sweating of palms of hands
- Sprained pain in right wrist, on motion
- Cramps in hands all night and trembling in afternoon, worse from lifting heavy weights

Symptoms *Better*
• Dry climate and weather
• Lying on painful side
• Sneezing
• Rubbing
• From drawing the limbs up
• While lying on the back in the dark and dry weather

The following symptoms generally accompany the above symptoms . . .

- It is generally suited to *children and women*
- The remedy is suited *to persons who are fatty, flabby and obese*
- Children whose head is too large, they *crave eggs and eat dirt,* and are prone to diarrhoea

- ✦ Children milestone are delayed especially walking and talking
- ✦ There is great sensitiveness to take cold
- ✦ *Profuse perspiration,* local and general, from slight exertion; *while sleeping wetting the pillow*
- ✦ Patient is very *apprehensive, forgetful* and has a variety of fears
- ✦ Sensation of coldness in general of single parts—head, stomach, feet and legs
- ✦ Periodicity of symptoms—commonly of 7 to 14 days
- ✦ *Enlarged glands*—Tonsils and other glands
- ✦ *Nostrils sore* and *ulcerated*
- ✦ Sour taste in mouth
- ✦ Craving of *indigestible things—chalk, coal, pencils*
- ✦ Frequent sour eructations, sour vomiting. *All discharges sour*
- ✦ Dislike of fat. May be aversion to milk
- ✦ *Loss of appetite when overworked*
- ✦ Menses *too early, too profuse, too long* with vertigo. *Milky white discharge*
- ✦ Painless hoarseness, shortness of breath on walking especially on going upstairs
- ✦ Aversion to open air
- ✦ Fever with night sweats, especially on head

Calcarea Phosphorica 30

4 pills three times daily for one month

Symptoms

- ✦ Shooting, tearing and aching type of rheumatic pain in all parts of body especially knees, loins and thumb

- ✦ Pain with stiffness, coldness, *numbness and crawling sensation*
- ✦ Pain become worse by any change of weather
- ✦ Buttocks, back and limbs fall asleep
- ✦ Weary when going upstairs. Cannot rise from seat. Staggering in old people when rising from a seat
- ✦ Pain in joints and bones excited or increased by every draft of cold damp air
- ✦ Rheumatism of cold weather, getting well in spring and the symptoms returning in autumn

Symptoms *Worse*
• Exposure to cold and damp weather
• Cold air
• Melting snow
• Changeable weather
• East winds
• Mental exertion
• Dinner
• After a meal, especially juicy fruits
• Motion

The following symptoms generally accompany the above symptom . . .

- ✦ For anaemic persons, especially *anaemic children* who are flabby, have cold extremities and feeble digestion
- ✦ Children—*emaciated, unable to stand, and slow in learning to walk*
- ✦ *Feels complaints more when thinking about them*
- ✦ *Numbness and crawling* are characteristic sensations

Symptoms *Better*
• In summer
• Warm, dry atmosphere
• Lying down
• Rest
• Passing wind

- Symptoms get worse by wet cold air and every *change of weather*
- Headache, *worse near the region of sutures*
- Glandular enlargement—swollen tonsils. *Adenoid growths*
- *Craving for bacon, ham, salted or smoked meat*
- *Much flatulence.* Flatulence temporarily relieved by sour eructations
- Pain in abdomen *at every attempt to eat*
- Diarrhoea from juicy fruits, during dentition *with fetid flatus*
- White discharge in females, like *white of egg*

Causticum 30

4 pills three times daily for one month

Symptoms

- It is mainly useful in chronic rheumatic, arthritic and paralytic affections
- Generally indicated by tearing, drawing pains in the muscular and fibrous tissues, with deformities about the joints, especially knee and shoulder joint
- Restlessness in night with tearing pain of joints
- Pains are severe, generally remain in one joint for a long time
- Joints are stiff

Symptoms *Worse*
• In dry cold wind
• In clear, fine weather
• Cold air
• From motion of carriage
• Expectoration
• Walking
• New moon
• After stools

- *Rheumatic tearing in limbs*
- Burning in joints
- Dull and tearing pain in hands and arm
- Rheumatism of the jaw with great stiffness
- Unsteadiness of *muscles of forearm* and hands
- Numbness, loss of sensation in hands
- Rheumatic pain of shoulders, cannot raise hand, painful stiffness between scapulae
- Pain in nape of neck as from bruises
- *Contracted tendons*
- Weak ankles, cannot walk without suffering
- Unsteady walking and easy falling
- *Restless legs at night.* Cannot find a position to lie still in bed for a moment at night
- Cracking and tension in knees, stiffness in hollow of knee
- Painful stiffness in the limbs through the hips, especially on rising from a seat or from a recumbent position
- Itching on the dorsum of feet

Symptoms *Better*
• By warmth, especially heat of bed
• In damp, wet weather
• Open air
• Stooping low
• Emission of flatus

The following symptoms generally accompany the above symptoms . . .

- Causticum patient is sad, hopeless, dark complexioned and *intensely sympathetic*
- *Burning, rawness* and *soreness* are characteristic
- General tendency of paralytic affection

- Restlessness at night and faint-like sinking of strength. Thus weakness progresses towards paralysis
- Paralysis of single parts—vocal cards, muscles of swallowing, of tongue, eyelids, face, bladder and extremities
- Dirty white sallow skin with warts especially on the face
- Symptoms worse on right side of body
- *Coryza with hoarseness*
- *Pimples and warts* on nose
- Aversion to sweets
- Thirst for cold water but aversion to drinking
- Menses cease at night, *flow only during day*
- *Hoarseness* with pain in chest and *loss of voice*
- Cough with *raw soreness of chest*
- Expectoration scanty, must be swallowed
- Cough with *pain in hip*, worse in evening, *better with drinking cold water*
- Difficulty of voice of singers and public speakers
- *Warts* large, bleeding easily, on tips of fingers and nose
- *Retention of urine*
- Bed wetting soon after falling asleep (during first sleep)
- Involuntary urine may also dribble while coughing or sneezing or after any excitement
- Constant mental stress, effects of shock or grief, any long standing worry

Lycopodium 30

4 pills three times daily for one month

Symptoms

- It is useful in chronic rheumatism and arthritis
- Rheumatic pain may occur in any of the joints of the body but knee and finger joints are commonly affected
- Numbness, drawing and tearing in limbs especially while at rest or at night
- Pain will often have started on right-side of the body and moved over to the left
- Spasmodic contraction and extension without pain
- Pains come and go suddenly
- Heaviness of arms
- Tearing in shoulder and elbow joints
- Tearing pain in joints with stiffness
- *Chronic gout,* with chalky deposits in joints with urinary trouble; red sand and clear urine
- Gout which affects especially the right side
- Pain in heel on treading as from a pebble
- Profuse sweat on the feet

Symptoms *Worse*

- From right to left
- From above downwards
- 4 to 8 p.m.
- At night
- From heat or warm room
- Hot air
- Warmth of bed
- Warm application (expect throat and stomach which are better from warm drinks)
- On beginning to move

- ✦ Hands and feet numb
- ✦ Swelling of feet, worse right side
- ✦ Cramps in calves and toes at night in bed
- ✦ Twitching and jerking

The following symptoms generally accompany the above symptoms . . .

- ✦ In nearly all cases where Lycopodium is the remedy, some evidence of urinary or digestive disturbance will be found
- ✦ Ailment develops gradually
- ✦ A *right-sided* remedy, complaints travel from right to left or from above downwards
- ✦ Symptoms are generally *worse* from *4 p.m. to 8 p.m*
- ✦ Its patient is generally lean, flatulent, wrinkled and *prematurely old*
- ✦ Carving for sweets and warm food and drinks
- ✦ Patient is *apprehensive, afraid to be alone,* spells or writes wrong words
- ✦ Although *hungry but eating ever so little (few bites) create fullness*
- ✦ Food tastes sour
- ✦ Blisters on tongue
- ✦ Abdomen is bloated, full due to accumulation of wind, coupled with rumbling, gurgling and distension
- ✦ Stool hard, difficult to expel

Symptoms *Better*
- From continued motion
- After midnight
- Stomach and throat complaint relieved by warm drink and food
- On getting cold
- In cool open air
- On being uncovered

- Dark, scanty urine, red sand in urine, frequency of urination increased at night
- Impotency in males

Rhododendron 30

4 pills three times daily for one month

Symptoms

- Well marked *rheumatic and gouty* symptoms
- It can affect *mainly small joints*
- Joints are red and swollen
- *Rheumatic tearing* in *all limbs,* especially right side
- Numbness and formication
- Rheumatic pain in bones in spots and they reappear by change of weather
- Pain in shoulders, arms and wrists
- Pain in limbs especially felt in the forearm and leg down to the fingers and toes
- Digging, drawing sprained pains in wrists
- Heaviness, weakness and tremors in hand
- Paralytic pain in right shoulder when resting open it, sometimes extending below elbow
- Heaviness in thighs. Pain in hips as if sprained
- *Cannot sleep unless legs are crossed*

Symptoms *Worse*
- Before a storm
- All symptoms reappear in rough weather
- Windy weather
- Wet cold weather
- Night
- Towards morning
- Rest
- Wine

- Gouty inflammation of great toe-joint with swelling and redness
- Acute and chronic gouty condition

The following symptoms generally accompany the above symptoms . . .

- Patient is gloomy, forgetful and afraid of thunderstorm
- All symptoms are worse before a storm, relieved when it breaks
- Pain in lower jaw and chin, better with *warmth* and *eating*
- Testicles, intensely painful to touch, drawn up, swollen and painful. Hydrocoele

Symptoms *Better*
- After a storm breaks
- Warmth
- Dry heat
- Exercise
- By eating
- From wrapping the head
- Immediately on starting to move

If there is no improvement after taking the above remedies then please consult a trained homoeopathic practitioner.

Acupressure

It can provide relief of symptomatic pain by stimulating circulation, calming nerves and activating the body's own painkilling agents. An experienced practitioner may treat all the symptoms of hands, wrist, fingers and shoulder.

Physiotherapy

A physiotherapist treats it by a combination of massage by low level electric stimulation and ultra sound rays. Massage and ultrasound stimulate the blood circulation along with relaxing the muscles and reducing tensions.

A few minutes of warm-up exercises before the beginning of work and regular tension-relieving exercises throughout the work during the day can have a positive, preventive effect.

Yoga

+ Yoga that relaxes the neck and back may be advisable. Avoid hand and neck stands, as well as positions that include arm twists, any of which could harm the already sensitive nerves

Herbal Therapy

+ Grate small piece of ginger and make an infusion with half a cup of hot water (not boiling). Dip a soft, folded cloth into the infusion and apply it to the affected area, cover it with a dry cloth to retain heat

Diet and Nutrition

+ Avoid high protein diet—because it inhibits the absorption of vitamin B6
+ Cut down on sugar and sweets in general
+ Ginger has been shown in studies to have anti-inflammatory properties
+ Sources of vitamin B like spinach, green peeper etc. are advisable

Juice Therapy

+ Pineapple juice
+ Pineapple + apple + ginger juice
+ Broccoli, garlic clove, carrots, green peeper juice
+ Ginger, carrots + apple juice

- Ginger, apple juice with water

Home Remedies

- The most effective treatment at home for reducing discomfort, pain and numbness of hand, fingers are *cold pack* and *exercise*
- Few ice cube wrapped in a towel can be applied on an affected area for about an hour at a time, 10 minutes on the area and 10 minutes off
- Opening and closing your fist a dozen or more times is an effective exercise
- With palm facing each other, press your fingertips together 20 times, rest, then repeat
- Holding your hands over your head, rotate them at the wrist clockwise for 20 seconds, then rotate the same anti-clockwise

Prevention

If your job demands repetitive hand or finger work, take the following precautions to prevent carpal tunnel syndrome:

- Avoid forward and backward bending at the wrist for extended periods because it stresses the nerves, so learn to keep your wrist and hand as straight as possible while in work
- Take frequent breaks and do exercises for your hands and wrists frequently
- If you work at a keyboard, use a wrist support to prevent unnatural bending
- Make sure that the desk and chair height are correct for your stature
- Finally if symptoms appear, get a professional advice

CHAPTER 8

Tendinitis

Tendon is a band of fibrous tissue that connects a muscle to a bone and transmits the force that the muscles exerts. Inflammation of a tendon is known as tendinitis; it usually occurs simultaneously with that of the sheath surrounding it (tenosynovitis).

Tendons are designed to withstand bending, stretching, and twisting. The cause is often unknown, but the condition mostly affects middle aged or older people after repeated slight strains or excessive unaccustomed activity. They can also inflame due to overuse, disease or injuries that results in torn fibers or other damage. Tendinitis generally heals in about two weeks, but it becomes chronic if sufferer doesn't give time to the tendon to heal. Healing is generally slow in case of diabetes, arthritis and gout.

The tendinitis most often affects tendons surrounding the shoulder and hip joints, those that bend the wrists and fingers and straighten the thumbs, the achilles tendons at the back of the heels and tendons behind the knees. 'Trigger-finger' is an example of tendinitis in which there is locking of one or more fingers in a bend-position. Normally when the muscle that bends the finger contracts, its tendon is pulled along its sheath, but inflammation of tendon prevents it from slipping back to allow straightening of the fingers.

Affected tendons are painful on movement and swollen due to inflammation and fluid accumulation.

Causes

- Repetitive stress—using the same joint for the same stressful movement again and again. This happens in sports and many type of office work and other situations
- *Weekend athletes*—who exercise occasionally rather than regularly
- Infection—Infection of the synovial-linning of the tendon by bacteria. It is common in the tendons of hands and forearms
- Injuries

Symptoms

- Tendons are painful on movement at or near a joint, especially around shoulder joint, wrist, heel (Achilles tendinitis), behind knee
- Swelling due to inflammation and accumulation of fluid
- Stiffness of joint tending to restriction of movement

Consult a Doctor if

+ Your pain doesn't subside within in a week or more
+ Extremely severe pain with swelling; you may have a ruptured tendon

Lab Investigations

+ X-ray—calcium deposit in the tendon may be seen on X-ray
+ X-ray to rule out any bone damage
+ MRI—It can help to determine the severity of damage to a tendon

Treatment and Management

+ The main aim of treatment is to restore movement of the joint without pain and to maintain strength in the surrounding muscles while giving time to the tissue to heal
+ Adequate rest is required
+ RICE program is recommended : rest, ice, compression and elevation. *(See page no. 6)*

Homoeopathy

Massage the affected area with *Arnica* or *Rhus tox.* ointment to relieve tenderness.

The following remedies are generally indicated in tendinitis.

Rhus Toxicodendron 30

4 pills three times daily for one month

Symptoms

- Hot, painful swelling of joint
- Tearing and drawing pain
- *Limbs stiff, paralysed sensation*
- Tenderness about knee joint
- Trembling after exertion
- Tingling in feet
- Loss of power in forearm and fingers
- Crawling sensation in the tips of fingers
- *Tearing pain in tendons, ligament and fasicae*
- Numbness after over work and exposure
- Soreness of condyles of bones
- Pains aching, sore, bruised, tearing, shooting with heaviness, lameness and stiffness
- *Sprains, strains, torn ligaments and tendinitis*

Symptoms *Worse*

- The cold fresh air is not tolerable
- Damp weather and after rains
- From sitting and rising from sitting position or first attempt to move
- Approach of storms
- At night, especially in bed
- After overwork and exposure
- From gardening
- Checked perspiration
- Injuries after lifting and over exertion

The following symptoms generally accompany the above symptoms . . .

- *Extreme restlessness* accompanies most symptoms. Cannot stay in one position, continued change of position
- Aching in bone with fever

- ✦ Tongue coated, except red triangular space at tip with great thirst
- ✦ Bitter taste in mouth
- ✦ Skin eruptions—red, swollen with intense itching
- ✦ Desire for milk
- ✦ Fever of typhoid character
- ✦ General or localised glandular swelling
- ✦ Trembling and palpitation of heart when siting still
- ✦ *Sensitive to open air,* putting the hand from under the bed-cover brings on cough

> **Symptoms *Better***
> - For external heat
> - Warm compresses
> - From warmth of bed
> - Continued movement
> - Change of position
> - Moving affected part
> - Rubbing
> - From stretching out limbs

Phytolacca 30

4 pills three times daily for one month

Symptoms

- ✦ It mainly acts well in chronic rheumatism
- ✦ A sore, bruised, aching feeling all over the body; he feels he must move, movement increases his pain and soreness
- ✦ Rheumatic pain, worse in the morning
- ✦ *Pains fly like electric shocks*
- ✦ Shooting, lancinating pain shifting rapidly
- ✦ Rheumatic swelling are hard, painful on touch and intensely hot
- ✦ Shooting pain in cardiac region alternating with pain in the right shoulder

- ✦ Shooting pain in right shoulder, with stiffness and inability to raise arm
- ✦ Pain on undersides of thighs
- ✦ *Aching of heels,* relieved by elevating feet
- ✦ Pain in the right knee in afternoon, worse in open air and damp weather
- ✦ Pain in legs, patient dreads to get up and move
- ✦ Pain like shocks
- ✦ Swelling in feet
- ✦ Pain in ankle and feet
- ✦ Neuralgic pain in big toes
- ✦ Rheumatism of fibrous and periosteal tissue

The following symptoms generally accompany the above symptoms . . .

- ✦ Aching, soreness, restlessness, weakness are guiding general symptoms
- ✦ Glandular swelling with heat and inflammation
- ✦ *Pain flying like electric shocks;* rapidly shifting pains
- ✦ *Increased secretion of tears*
- ✦ Right-sided remedy especially in throat

Symptoms *Worse*

- In the morning on rising
- Sensitive to electric changes
- Effects of a wetting, when it rains
- Exposure to damp, cold weather
- Night
- Motion
- On the right side
- Hot drinks (especially in throat problem)

Symptoms *Better*

- Warmth
- Dry weather
- Rest

- *Children bite teeth or gums together* during teething
- *Throat feels rough, narrow,* hot. *Tonsils swollen*
- *Shooting pain into the ears on swallowing.* Cannot swallow anything hot
- Throat feels very hot, pain at root of tongue extending to ear
- Urine scanty and suppressed with pain in kidney region
- *Breast hard swollen and very sensitives*
- Disposition to boils

Rhododendron 30
4 pills three times daily for one month

Symptoms
- Well marked *rheumatic and gouty* symptoms
- It can affect *mainly small joints*
- Joints are red and swollen
- *Rheumatic tearing* in *all limbs,* especially on the right side
- Numbness and formication
- Rheumatic pain in bones in spots and they reappear by change of weather
- Pain in shoulders, arms and wrists
- Pain in limbs especially felt in the forearm and leg down to the fingers and toes
- Digging, drawing spanned pains in wrists

Symptoms *Worse*
• Before a storm
• All symptoms reappear in rough weather
• Windy weather
• Wet cold weather
• Night
• Towards morning
• Rest
• Wine

- Heaviness, weakness and tremors in hand
- Paralytic pain in right shoulder when resting open it, sometimes extending below elbow
- Heaviness in thighs. Pain in hips as it sprained
- *Cannot sleep unless legs are crossed*
- Gouty inflammation of great toe-joint with swelling and redness
- Acute and chronic gouty conditions

Symptoms *Better*
• After a storm breaks
• Warmth
• Dry heat
• Exercise
• By eating
• From wrapping the head
• Immediately on when starting to move

The following symptoms generally accompany the above symptoms . . .

- Patient is gloomy, forgetful and afraid during thunderstorms
- All symptoms worse before a storm, relieved when it breaks
- Pain in lower jaw and chin, better with *warmth* and *eating*
- Testicles, intensely painful to touch, drawn up, swollen and painful. Hydrocoele

Bryonia Alba 30
4 pills three times daily for one month

Symptoms
- *Joint red, hot, swollen with stitches and tearing*
- Knees stint and painful
- Every spot is painful on pressure
- During sprain and strain, joint is painful and swollen, distended with fluid with great stiffness

Tendinitis

- Weariness and heaviness in all limbs and stiffness
- Swelling of elbow extending as far as middle of upper arm and of forearm
- Swollen sensation in joints of finger on writing or taking hold of anything with pain
- Heaviness and weakness of legs while walking and on standing
- Stitching pain in hip joint extending to knees
- Weariness of thigh worse while ascending stairs; better when descending
- *Constant motion of left arm and leg*

The following symptoms generally accompany the above symptoms . . .

- *Dryness of all mucous membranes* like lips, mouth, throat, nose, chest, digestive tract
- *Excessive thirst.* Drinks large quantity of cold water
- Symptom develop slowly
- Patient is irritable
- Patient wants to be left alone, wants to go home even when at home
- Delirium—talks of business

Symptoms *Worse*

- From least motion and touch, caused by jar, by change of position, by any effort to talk, to cough, even by moving eye balls and by winking
- Hot weather after a cold spell and warmth
- Intolerance of heat
- After eating
- Exertion
- Suppressed perspiration
- 9 p.m.
- Morning

- ✦ Complaints which come on *after humiliation and anger*
- ✦ Right-sided complaints
- ✦ Physical weakness
- ✦ Nausea and faintness when rising up
- ✦ Pressure in stomach after eating, as of a stone
- ✦ Bursting, splitting headache
- ✦ Breast hot and painful, hard
- ✦ Chest painful, while coughing
- ✦ Constipation; *stool hard, dry, dark, as if burnt*
- ✦ *Stitches* and stiffness in small of back
- ✦ Cough, dry, spasmodic with gagging and vomiting, after eating and drinking

Symptoms *Better*
- Hard pressure and rest
- Lying on the painful side
- From perspiring
- Cold things, cold air, cold water
- Darkened room

Belladonna 30
4 pills three times daily for one month

Symptoms
- ✦ It is a good remedy in acute and chronic rheumatism of an inflammatory nature
- ✦ Joints swollen, red and shining
- ✦ Shooting, tearing, aching, throbbing or bruise-like pain
- ✦ *Pain comes suddenly and disappears suddenly*
- ✦ Symptoms prefer right side
- ✦ Shifting rheumatic pains means pain changes position from one joint to another
- ✦ Patient is extremely sensitive to touch or jar
- ✦ Shooting pain along limbs

Tendinitis

- Jerking limbs
- Involuntary limping
- Pain with redness of eyes and face
- *Cold extremities*
- Oppressive tearing pain in shoulders
- Paralytic twitching of arms with red swelling of hands and arms
- Paralytic feeling and weakness of whole left arm
- Tearing in middle joint of right index finger or in proximal joint of left middle finger
- Unsteady while walking
- Cutting stitches in outer muscles of right thigh, just above the knee, only when sitting
- Pain in thighs and legs as if caries
- When rising from bed, legs unable to carry the body weight and he sinks to the ground
- Stitches in hip joint, as if beaten

Symptoms *Worse*
• In the afternoon, after 3 p.m.
• At night, especially after midnight
• Touching the affected part
• Jar
• Noise
• Draught of air
• Lying down
• Cold
• Uncovering head
• Sudden changes from warm to cold weather
• In hot weather
• Hot sun
• While looking at bright, shining object
• While drinking

The following symptoms generally accompany the above symptoms . . .

- Sudden and violent onset of disease which also disappears suddenly. *Pains come on suddenly and disappear suddenly*
- For inflammatory condition with heat, redness, throbbing and burning

- ✦ Complaints from cold, dry wind, especially from exposure of head to cold wind or getting head wet
- ✦ *Great children remedy*
- ✦ Redness of toes, eyes and of inflamed part
- ✦ Oversensitive to pain, worse from slight touch, (worse from pressure of cloth, bed covering slight movement and least jar)
- ✦ Right sided remedy— Symptoms occur largely on the right side
- ✦ Great thirst for cold water but *anxiety or fear of drinking*
- ✦ Throat feels constricted, difficulty in deglutition. Tonsils enlarged
- ✦ Retension of urine, *frequent and profuse urination*
- ✦ Menses too early, too profuse and very offensive and hot
- ✦ Ticking, short, dry cough, worse at night
- ✦ Glands *swollen, tender,* red. *Boils*
- ✦ Alternate redness and paleness of skin

Symptoms *Better*
• Walking in open air
• When standing up after sitting
• While leaving the head against something
• Sitting erect
• Warm application (except in headache)
• Wrapping up
• In a warm room

Following an analysis of overall situation you can take remedies that may relieve pain and other symptoms. If there is no improvement after taking remedies then please consult a trained homoeopathic practitioner.

Physiotherapy

- Rest the injured tendon
- Strengthening near muscles group
- Maintain overall muscle tone
- Ultrasonic rays
- Once you heal properly, you may work into easy stretching exercises, done several times a day

Herbal Therapy

- White willow (Salix alba) is taken orally
- Pineapple is sometimes taken orally for reducing inflammation in soft tissues

Home Remedies

- Remind yourself of RICE—rest, ice, compression and elevation. *(See page no. 7)*
- In chronic case apply alternating hot and cold compression to the sore area. Soak one wash cloth in hot water and another in cold. Place warm cloth over the affected area for 3 minutes; follow with the cold cloth for 30 seconds. Alternate them twice and end with the cold cloth. Do this once or twice a day
- Once your tendinitis heals, you should devise a weight lifting program for yourself that gradually rebuilds the weakened muscles. Don't do it excessively, putting too much strain on the muscles too soon may cause the tendon to become inflamed again

Prevention

✦ For prevention of tendonitis warm up before any repetitive stress movement and take frequent breaks during repetitive stress movement

✦ Include warm ups, cool downs, and stretches in your exercise routine

Chapter 9

Dislocation

Dislocation cannot occur without damage to the protective ligament or joint capsule. Usually the capsule and one or more ligaments are torn causing escape of bone through the vent. *(See figure 9.1).*

Causes

- Due to injury—Injury is the commonest cause of dislocation at almost all joints
- Some people suffer repeated dislocations after minor injuries without any apparent reason
- Articular surface forming a joint may be destroyed by an infection

- The ligaments may be damaged due to some disease; it causes dislocation of joint without any injury
- Congenital disorder is a defect where a joint is dislocated at birth, e.g., congenital dislocation of the hip

Patho-anatomy of dislocations

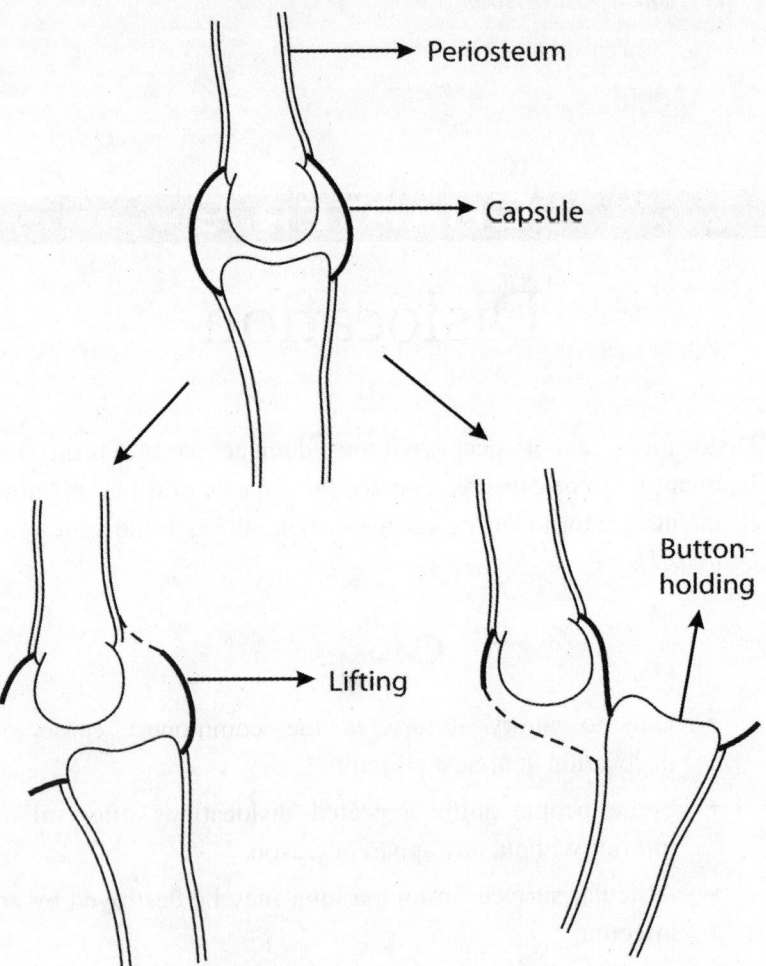

Fig. 9.1 *Showing Dislocation*

Symptoms

- Deformity of the area
- Pain—dislocations are very painful
- Swelling in the joint region
- Retardation of movement because of severe pain and muscle spasm
- Shortening of the limb occurs in most dislocations
- Tenderness at the joint

Consult A Doctor If

+ There is pain, swelling and tenderness in the joint area after an injury; it may be sprain or strain
+ Loss of movement of joint

Lab Investigations

+ Most dislocations are obvious from the symptoms
+ X-ray is done to confirm the dislocation

Treatment and Management

+ The dislocated joints are manipulated into their correct position
+ The joint is immobilised by bandaging or with a splint to prevent further discomfort. The joint usually recovers its normal function in several weeks

Homoeopathy

The following remedies are usually indicated in dislocation:

Calcarea Carbonica 30

4 pills three times daily for one month

Symptoms

It is a useful remedy for rheumatoid arthritis, chronic and acute muscular rheumatism, gouty nodosities

- Rheumatic pains, after getting wet
- Sharp sticking pain, as if parts were sprained
- *Cold, damp feet,* feels as if damp stockings were worn
- Pains are shooting, cutting or tearing, sometimes confined to small spots
- Pains are associated with cramps, contraction, stiffness and weakness all over body
- Cold knees
- Cramp in calves
- Sour foot sweat
- Swelling of joints, especially knee
- Inflammation of hip joints which is painfully sore
- Burning of soles of feet which feels cold and dead at night
- Weakness in the muscles of thigh in morning, on beginning to walk, with stiffness, *worse while ascending stairs or any height*

Symptoms *Worse*
• From exertion, mental or physical
• Ascending
• Cold in every form
• Washing, moist air, wet weather
• During full moon
• Standing
• After eating
• In the evening, after midnight

- Pain in calves on stepping, on touch and on bending foot
- *Soles of feet raw*
- Ankles weary, feels as if dislocated
- Tearing in muscles
- Rheumatoid arthritis of finger joints with swelling and arthritic nodosities on hand and finger joints
- Pain in upper arm, as if beaten
- Sweating of palms of hands
- Sprained pain in right wrist, on motion
- Cramps in hands all night and trembling in afternoon, worse from lifting heavy weights

Symptoms *Better*
• Dry climate and weather
• Lying on painful side
• Sneezing
• Rubbing
• From drawing the limbs up
• While lying on the back in the dark and dry weather

The following symptoms generally accompany the above symptoms . . .

- It is generally suited to *children and women*
- The remedy is suited *to persons who are fatty, flabby and obese*
- Children whose head is too large, they *crave eggs and eat dirt,* and are prone to diarrhoea
- Children milestone are delayed especially walking and talking
- There is great sensitiveness to take cold
- *Profuse perspiration,* local and general, from slight exertion; *while sleeping wetting the pillow*
- Patient is very *apprehensive, forgetful* and cries often

- Sensation of coldness in general of single parts—head, stomach, feet and legs
- Periodicity of symptoms—commonly of 7 to 14 days
- *Enlarged glands*—Tonsils and other glands
- *Nostrils sore* and *uncreated*
- Sour taste in mouth
- Craving of *indigestible things—chalk, coal, pencils*
- Frequent sour eructations, sour vomiting. *All discharges sour*
- Dislike of fat. May be aversion to milk
- *Loss of appetite when overworked*
- Menses *too early, too profuse, too long* with vertigo. *Milky white discharge*
- Painless hoarseness, shortness of breath on walking especially on going upstairs
- Aversion to open air
- Fever with night sweats, especially on head

Causticum 30

4 pills three times daily for one month

Symptoms

- It is mainly useful in chronic rheumatic, arthritic and paralytic affections
- Generally indicated by tearing, drawing pains in the muscular and fibrous tissues, with deformities about the joints, especially knee and shoulder joint
- Restlessness in night with tearing pain of joints
- Pains are severe, generally they remain in one joint for a long time

Dislocation

- Joints are stiff
- *Rheumatic tearing in limbs*
- Burning in joints
- Dull and tearing pain in hands and arm
- Rheumatism of the jaw with great stiffness
- Unsteadiness of *muscles of forearm* and hands
- Numbness, loss of sensation in hands
- Rheumatic pain of shoulders, cannot raise hand, painful stiffness between scapulae
- Pain in nape of neck as from bruises
- *Contracted tendons*
- Weak ankles, cannot walk without suffering
- Unsteady walking and easy falling
- *Restless legs at night*. Cannot find a position to lie still in bed for a moment at night
- Cracking and tension in knees, stiffness in the hollow of knee
- Painful stiffness in the limbs through the hips, especially on rising from a seat or from a recumbent position
- Itching on the dorsum of feet

Symptoms *Worse*
• In dry cold wind
• In clear, fine weather
• Cold air
• From motion of carriage
• Expectoration
• Walking
• New moon
• After stools

Symptoms *Better*
• By warmth, especially heat of bed
• In damp, wet weather
• Open air
• By stooping low
• Emission of flatus

The following symptoms generally accompany the above symptoms . . .

- Causticum patient is sad, hopeless, dark complexioned *intensely sympathetic*
- *Burning, rawness* and *soreness* are characteristic
- General tendency of paralytic affection
- Restlessness at night and faint-like sinking of strength. Thus weakness progresses towards paralysis
- Paralysis of single parts—vocal cards, muscles of swallowing, of tongue, eyelids, face, bladder and extremities
- Dirty white sallow skin with warts especially on the face
- Symptoms worse on right side of body
- *Coryza with hoarseness*
- *Pimples and warts* on nose
- Aversion to sweets
- Thirst for cold water but aversion to drinking
- Menses cease at night, *flow only during day*
- *Hoarseness* with pain in chest and *loss of voice*
- Cough with *raw soreness of chest*
- Expectoration scanty, must be swallowed
- Cough with *pain in hip*, worse in evening, *better with drinking cold water*
- Difficulty of voice of singers and public speakers
- *Warts* large, bleed easily, on tips of fingers and nose
- *Retention of urine*
- Bed wetting soon after falling asleep (during first sleep)
- Involuntary urine may also dribble while coughing or sneezing or after any excitement

- Constant mental stress, effects of shock or grief, any long standing worry

Arnica Montana 30
4 pills three times daily for one month

Symptoms

- Rheumatism of muscular and tendinous tissue, especially of hip, back and shoulders
- It is suited to cases when any injury, however remote, seems to have caused the present trouble. *After traumatic injury*
- A muscular tonic
- Limbs and body aches as if beaten; joints as if sprained
- *Sore, lame and bruised feeling*
- Sharp, shooting, paralytic or sprained pains which quickly change place
- *Gouty affections.* Great fear at being touched or approached
- Sore, tender, red swelling of the joints in gout, particularly of knee joint
- Gout with arthritic pains in the feet and the big toe as if sprained
- In arthritis especially hip joint affected
- Rheumatism begins low down and works up
- Cannot walk erect, on account of bruised pain in pelvic region

Symptoms Worse
• Least touch
• Motion
• Rest
• Wine
• Damp cold
• In the evening
• From speaking
• Blowing nose
• Almost any noise
• Lying on the injured part
• From over exertion
• Alcohol
• Old age

- ✦ Paralytic pains in all joints during motion
- ✦ Knee bends suddenly when walking, stitches when touched
- ✦ Twitching pain from left shoulder joint to middle finger
- ✦ Pain in back and limbs, as if bruised
- ✦ Deathly coldness of forearms
- ✦ Everything on which he lies seems too hard
- ✦ Soreness after over-exertion
- ✦ Cracking in the right wrist when the hand is moved, as if dislocated
- ✦ During *Sprains* and *Strains* ligaments torn with swelling which is most prominent. Bruising and inflammation of the soft tissue around the joint
- ✦ When muscles or soft tissues are black and blue

Symptoms *Better*
• Lying down
• Warmth
• Rubbing and wrapping up warmly
• Long walk in cold weather
• Out stretched
• Changing position

Following symptoms generally accompany the above symptoms . . .

- ✦ Produces conditions similar to those resulting from injuries, falls, blows, contusions
- ✦ Especially suited to cases when any injury occurs. *After any traumatic injuries*
- ✦ Remote effects of injuries even though it was received years ago
- ✦ Whole body feels sore and *bruised, lame* and does not want to be approached, touched or jarred
- ✦ It promotes healing, reduces swelling, prevents pus formation

- ✦ It is very effective in bleeding of any kind
- ✦ *Head hot with cold body*
- ✦ Fetid breath
- ✦ Diarrhoea offensive any bloody
- ✦ *Violent spasmodic cough with facial herpes*
- ✦ Skin *black and blue*. Multiple small boils very painful. Acne characterised by *symmetry in distribution*
- ✦ *Aids recovery after an operation*

Rhus Toxicodendron 30

4 pills three times daily for one month

Symptoms

- ✦ Hot, painful swelling of joint
- ✦ Tearing and drawing pain
- ✦ *Limbs stiff, paralysed sensation*
- ✦ Tenderness about knee joint
- ✦ Trembling after exertion
- ✦ Tingling in feet
- ✦ Loss of power in forearm and fingers
- ✦ Crawling sensation in the tips of fingers
- ✦ *Tearing pain in tendons, ligament and fasciae*
- ✦ Numbness after over work and exposure
- ✦ Soreness of condyles of bones
- ✦ Pains aching, sore, bruised, tearing, shooting with heaviness, lameness and stiffness

Symptoms Worse

- The cold fresh air is not tolerable
- Damp weather and after rains
- From sitting and rising from sitting position or first attempt to move
- Approach of storms
- At night, especially in bed
- After overwork and exposure
- From gardening
- Checked perspiration
- Injuries after lifting and overexertion

- *Sprains, strains, torn ligaments and tendinitis*

The following symptoms generally accompany the above symptoms . . .

- *Extreme restlessness* accompanies most symptoms. Cannot stay in one position, continued changes of position
- Aching in bone with fever
- Tongue coated, except red triangular space at tip with great thirst
- Bitter taste in mouth
- Skin eruptions—red, swollen with intense itching
- Desire for milk
- Fever of typhoid character
- General or localised glandular swelling
- Trembling and palpitation of heart when siting still
- *Sensitive to open air,* putting the hand from under the bedcover brings on cough

Symptoms *Better*
• From external heat
• Warm compresses
• From warmth of bed
• Continued movement
• Change of position
• Moving the affected part
• Rubbing
• From stretching out limbs

Belladonna 30

4 pills three times daily for one month

Symptoms

- It is a good remedy in acute and chronic rheumatism of an inflammatory nature
- Joints swollen, red and shining
- Shooting, tearing, aching, throbbing or bruise-like pain

Dislocation

- *Pain comes suddenly and disappear suddenly*
- Symptoms prefer right side
- Shifting rheumatic pains means pain changes position from one joint to another
- Patient is extremely sensitive to touch or jar
- Shooting pain along limbs
- Jerking limbs
- Involuntary limping
- Pain with redness of eyes and face
- *Cold extremities*
- Pressive tearing pain in shoulders
- Paralytic twitching of arms with red swelling of hands and arms
- Paralytic feeling and weakness of whole left arm
- Tearing in middle joint of right index finger or in proximal joint of left middle finger
- Unsteady while walking
- Cutting stitches in outer muscles of right thigh, just above the knee, only when sitting
- Pain in thighs and legs as if caries
- When rising from bed, legs unable to carry the body weight and the patient sinks to the ground

Symptoms *Worse*

- In the afternoon, after 3 p.m.
- At night, especially after midnight
- Touching the affected part
- Jar
- Noise
- Draught of air
- Lying down
- Cold
- By uncovering the head
- Sudden changes from warm to cold weather
- In hot weather
- Hot sun
- While looking at bright, shining objects
- While drinking

✦ Stitches in hip joint, as if beaten

The following symptoms generally accompany the above symptoms . . .

✦ Sudden and violent onset of disease which also disappears suddenly. *Pains come on suddenly and disappear suddenly*

✦ For inflammatory condition with heat, redness, throbbing and burning

✦ Complaints from cold, dry wind, especially from exposure of head to cold wind or getting head wet

✦ *Great children remedy*

✦ Redness of toes, eyes and of inflamed part

✦ Oversensitive to pain worse from slight touch, (worse from pressure of cloth, bed covering) slight movement and least jar

✦ Right sided remedy—Symptoms occur largely on the right side

✦ Great thirst for cold water but *anxiety or fear of drinking*

✦ Throat feels constricted, difficulty in deglutition. Tonsils enlarged

✦ Retention of urine, *frequent and profuse urination*

✦ Menses too early, too profuse and very offensive and hot

✦ Ticking, short, dry cough, worse at night

✦ Glands *swollen, tender,* red. *Boils*

✦ Alternate redness and paleness of skin

Symptoms *Better*
• Walking in the open air
• When standing up after sitting
• While leaning the head against something
• Sitting erect
• Warm application (except in headache)
• Wrapping up
• In a warm room

Bryonia Alba 30
4 pills three times daily for one month

Symptoms

- *Joint red, hot, swollen with stitches and tearing*
- Knees stint and painful
- Every spot is painful on pressure
- During sprain and strain, joint in painful and swollen, distended with fluid with great stiffness
- Weariness and heaviness in all limbs and stiffness
- Swelling of elbow extending as far as middle of upper arm and of forearm
- Swollen sensation in joints of finger on writing or taking hold of anything with pain
- Heaviness and weakness of legs while walking and on standing
- Stitching pain in hip joint extending to knees
- Weariness of thigh worse while ascending stairs, better when descending
- *Constant motion of left arm and leg*

Symptoms *Worse*

- From least motion and touch, caused by jar, by change of position, by any effort to talk, to cough, even by moving eye balls and by winking
- Hot weather after a cold spell and warmth
- Intolerance of heat
- After eating
- Exertion
- Suppressed perspiration
- 9 p.m.
- Morning

The following symptoms generally accompany the above symptoms...

- *Dryness of all mucous membranes* like lips, mouth, throat, nose, chest, digestive tract

- *Excessive thirst.* Drinks large quantity of cold water
- Symptom develop slowly
- Patient is irritable
- Patient wants to be left alone, wants to go home even when at home
- Delirium—talks of business
- Complaints which come on *after humiliation and anger*
- Right-sided complaints
- Physical weakness
- Nausea and faintness when rising up
- Pressure in stomach after eating, as of a stone
- Bursting, splitting headache
- Breast hot and painful, hard
- Chest painful, while coughing
- Constipation, *stool hard, dry, dark, as if burnt*
- *Stitches* and stiffness in small of back
- Cough, dry, spasmodic with gagging and vomiting, after eating and drinking

Symptoms *Better*
• Hard pressure and rest
• Lying on painful side
• From perspiring
• Cold things, cold air, cold water
• Darkened room

Ruta Graveolens 30

4 pills three times daily for one month

Symptoms

- It acts upon bone, joints producing symptoms of a rheumatic nature
- For bruises that occurs on bone, e.g. chin, elbow, skull

- ✦ Pain is felt on surface of bone, particularly places where tendons are attached to the bone
- ✦ There is bruised pain all over the body, as after a fall, worse in limbs, spine and joints
- ✦ Especially in *sprains and strains* after injury when *Arnica* and *Rhus tox.* do not help
- ✦ Tendon or ligament that have been torn or wrenched
- ✦ Pain feels closer to the bone and can be associated with hard swelling where the tendon is attached to the bone
- ✦ Pain and stiffness in *wrist* and hands
- ✦ Tearing in right wrist, worse motion; pain in left wrist as if broken
- ✦ Bursa and ganglion of wrist
- ✦ *Veins of hands swell after eating. Fingers distorted*
- ✦ Wrenching pain in shoulder joints when the arms are allowed to hang down or when resting on them
- ✦ Pain between scapulae in the afternoon
- ✦ Tension and pressure in shoulders with stiffness in the morning
- ✦ *Thighs pain when stretching the limbs;* on rising from a seats, thighs and hips so weak, they are unable to support body weight so that the patient falls back on the seat

Symptoms *Worse*

- Lying down especially lying on painful part
- From cold
- Cold damp weather
- Rest
- Over-excretion
- Sitting or rising from a seat
- Lifting
- On stooping
- Beginning to move

Symptoms *Better*

- Dry warm weather
- Warmth
- Moving about

- Aching pain in tendo-achilles
- *Lameness and pain in ankle* with puffy swelling
- Hamstring feels shortened
- *Tendons sore;* working leaves patient weary and weak
- Pain in bones of feet and ankles. Pain in them does not permit to step heavily
- In *Tennis elbow* pain sore, bruised with lameness, worse from exercise

The following symptoms generally accompany the above symptoms...

- Feeling of intense lassitude, weakness and despair
- Restless, changes position frequently when lying
- All parts of body painful as if bruised
- Eyes painful with blurred vision from fine work like sewing or reading. Eyes red, hot and painful
- Difficult stool
- Prolapus ani
- Even after urination constant urging to urinate, feels bladder full
- Backache relieved by lying flat on the back

Pulsatilla 30
4 pills three times daily for one month

Symptoms

- Drawing, tearing pains in joints with swelling and redness, especially hips, knees, elbows and small joints of hand and feet
- The *pains shift* rapidly *from one part to another*
- Can hardly give symptoms and starts crying

- ✦ Rheumatic pains are so severe that the patient is compelled to move slowly, as easy motion relieves the pain
- ✦ Drawing, tensive pain in thighs and legs with restlessness and *chilliness*
- ✦ *Pain in limbs*, tensive pain, *letting up with a snap*
- ✦ Pain appears in a part, increase to a climax and then disappear suddenly from the part
- ✦ Pain in limbs in the morning in bed on waking with stiffness
- ✦ Hip-joint painful
- ✦ Knees swollen, with tearing, drawing pains
- ✦ Boring pain in heels like pricking of nails towards evening, *suffering worse from letting the affected limb hang down*
- ✦ Feet red inflamed and swollen
- ✦ Numbness around elbow
- ✦ Tearing in the shoulder joint obliging him to bend arms, extend intermittently to wrists and fingers
- ✦ Legs feel heavy and weary
- ✦ Nervousness, intensely felt about the ankles

Symptoms *Worse*

- From heat
- Rich fat food
- After eating
- In warm close room
- In the evening
- At twilight
- Lying on left or on the painless side
- When allowing feet to hang down
- When beginning to move
- On being seated or flexing (back)

Symptoms *Better*

- Cool open air
- Slow motion
- Cold application
- Cold food and drink
- Lying on the painful side
- Pressure or tying up tightly especially in head
- Rest

The following symptoms generally accompany the above symptoms . . .

- Very often indicated in the later, established stage of illness
- It is pre-eminently a female remedy, especially for mild, gentle, sad, crying, readily *weeps when talking, changeable,* contradictory
- Feels better by consolation
- The patient is chilly but she *feels better in open air and seeks the open air*
- Dry mouth but absence of thirst with nearly all complaints
- *Secretion* from all mucous membranes are *thick, bland and yellowish-green*
- *Symptoms ever changing*—no two stools, no two attacks alike; very well one hour, very miserable the next
- Pains *rapidly shifting* from one part to another
- Eyes inflammed and agglutinated, styes
- Cracks in middle of lower lips. *Yellow or white tongue*, covered with a tenacious mucous
- Desire for rich and fatty food, which leads to indigestion
- Dry cough in the evening and at night, must sit up in bed to get relief and loose cough in the morning. Pressure upon the chest and soreness
- Menses too late, scanty or suppressed
- Useful remedy to begin the treatment in a chronic case

Kali Iodide 30

4 pills three times daily for one month

Symptoms

- Rheumatic pain at night and in damp weather
- *Rheumatism of knee with effusion*

- ✦ Severe bone pains. Gnawing pain in left leg. Bones are sensitive to touch especially shin bone (leg bone)
- ✦ Contractions of joints
- ✦ Pain is hips causes limping when walking
- ✦ Gout affecting every joint with an indication that hepatic region is painful on touch
- ✦ Sensation as if small insects were crawling on the skin of lower extremities when sitting, better lying down
- ✦ Rheumatism in *neck, back,* feet especially heels and soles worse with cold and wet

Symptoms *Worse*
• Warm clothing
• Warm room
• At night
• Damp, wet weather
• Touch
• At rest
• Lying on painful side or on back

Symptoms *Better*
• Open air (walking in open air feels no fatigue)
• Motion

The following symptoms generally accompany the above symptoms . . .

- ✦ It acts prominently on fibrous and connective tissues, producing infiltration oedema
- ✦ *Glandular swelling*
- ✦ Emaciation and weakness
- ✦ Headache at *sides* and *root of nose*
- ✦ Profuse, *acrid, hot, watery, thin* discharge from nose
- ✦ Saliva increased, cold food and drink, especially milk, increases the suffering
- ✦ *Larynx feel raw.* Awakes choking. *Expectoration like soap-suds, greenish*
- ✦ Pimples with red tip

Sulphur 30

4 pills twice daily for fifteen days

Symptoms

- Rheumatic and arthritic complaints due to suppression of any skin disease
- *Painful stiffness* is main symptoms, with or without effusion
- For preventing gouty diathesis there is no better remedy than *Sulphur*
- One of the leading remedy for synovitis
- *Hot, sweaty hands*
- Trembling of hands
- Sprained pain in wrist
- Pain in left shoulder as if joint is dislocated
- Jerking in deltoid
- Drawing pain in shoulder and arms
- Swelling in fingers in the morning, sticking in tips at night; of flexure surface of right middle finger
- *Stooping shoulders*, cannot walk erect
- Tearing above the nail of left ring finger, worse in the evening

Symptoms *Worse*

- At rest
- Around 11 a.m.
- In the morning
- At night
- Warmth of bed
- When standing
- Washing and bathing
- From alcoholic stimulants
- From weather changes
- Periodically

Symptoms *Better*

- Dry, warm weather
- In open air
- Lying on right side
- From drawing up the affected limbs

Dislocation

- Sharp drawing, shooting and stitches here and there
- Pains seem to ascend, is worse in mid-summer heat, on clear and cloudless days
- Sweat in armpits which smells like garlic
- Stiffness of knees and ankles
- *Burning in soles and hands at night*
- Weakness of thighs and legs
- Tearing extending into middle of thigh, worse standing and on ascending stairs
- Tearing through knee extending to feet when walking and sitting
- Sprained wrenching pain in joints with cracking and stiffness, particularly in knees and shoulders
- Sudden cramp-like, painful jerking about the hip joints with stiffness
- Tension, pain in the joint on walking
- Tension in hollow of knees, as if too short, on stepping
- Inclination to cramp on stretching out feet
- Rheumatic gout with itching
- Swelling and inflammation of big toe with pain

The following symptoms generally accompany the above symptoms . . .

- Burning everywhere in the body especially head, palm and sole
- *Dirty, filthy people,* prone to skin disease, dry and hard hair and skin
- Children—*cannot bear to be washed or bathed*
- Aversion of being bathed

- *When carefully selected remedies fail to produce a favourable effect,* especially in acute disease
- Itching eruption on the skin. Scratching is followed by burning
- *Standing is the worse position* for patients, they cannot stand
- *Complaints are relapsing*—the patient seems to get almost well but the disease returns
- Redness of all orifices (lips, ears, eyelids, nostrils, anus, urethra etc.) as if pressed full of blood
- Discharges are offensive in character
- The discharges both of urine and faeces is painful to parts over which it passes; *parts around anus red, excoriated.* All the orifices of the body are very red
- Milk disagrees, craving for sugar, sweets and tatty food
- *Great acidity* and sour eructations
- *Diarrhoea,* painless, *driving out of bed early in the morning*
- Weak, empty gone feeling and faints about 11 a.m.

If there is no improvement after taking these remedies then please consult a trained homoeopathic physician.

Chapter 10

Bunions

A bunion is an unnatural bump or bend in the bone that forms on the ball of the foot out the base of big toe. The big toe is pushed towards the other toes and the joint protrudes on the inner side of the foot. If same thing happens on the little toe than condition is known as *bunionette*.

Bunions generally affect both feet. Women are more prone to the condition than men. Bunions usually develops due to continuous sideways pressure on the big toe from tight fitting shoes. First bursitis develops over the joint, followed by overgrowth of the bone and distortion of the joint. Bunions occurs at the joint where the toe bends in normal walking. They generally don't affect walking but they can be extremely painful. (*See figure 10.1*).

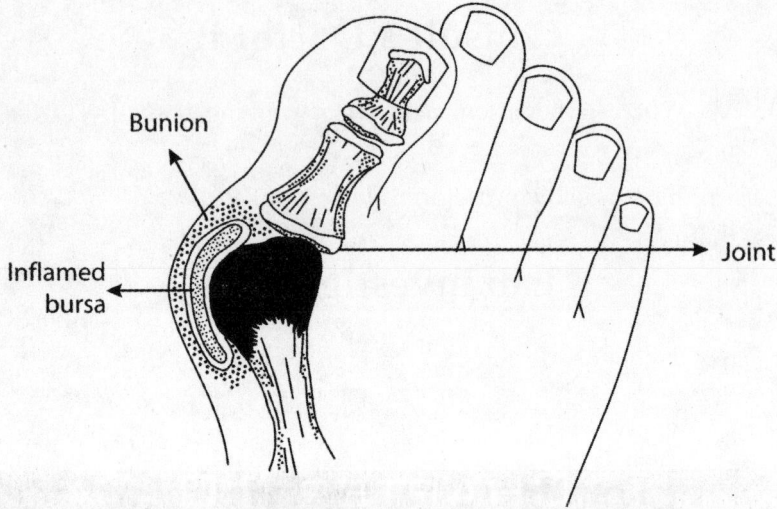

Fig. 10.1 *Showing Bunion, Knobby Protrusion of Large Joint of the Big Toe*

Causes

- ✦ Tight and poorly fitting shoes especially high heeled, pointed shoe
- ✦ It may be hereditary
- ✦ It occurs along with other problems associated with weak or poor foot structure, and with corns and calluses; bone spurs, and bursitis
- ✦ It can develop with arthritis

Symptoms

- Protrusion of the joint on the inner side of the foot, sometimes with hardened skin or a callus
- Swelling, pain, redness or tenderness at the base of big toe and in the ball of the foot

Consult a Doctor if

✦ There is persistent pain when walking normally in flat-soled foot
✦ Foot is showing deformity in shape

Lab investigations

✦ Generally detected by the unusual shape of the toe
✦ X-ray for confirmation and severity of the deformity

Treatment and Management

When bunions develop we first try to reduce pain and discomfort then we try to prevent recurrence.

If bunion is diagnosed early and there is no pain, then wearing well-made, well-fitting shoes may prevent further complications.

Homoeopathy

The following remedies are commonly used in Bunions:

Silica 30
4 pills three times daily for one month

Symptoms

✦ Mainly useful for the treatment of chronic rheumatism and arthritis
✦ Bruised pain in whole body, in the morning before walking, better while rising
✦ Bruised pain in all muscles of body
✦ Loss of power in legs

- Heaviness and weariness of lower limbs
- Pain in knee, as if tightly bound
- Calves tense and contracted
- Sole sores
- Soreness in feet
- Pain in great toes so that the patient can scarcely step on them
- Cramps in calves and soles
- *Icy cold and sweaty feet*
- Pain with weakness of joints, worse upper extremities of the ankle joint
- Biting pain in the hip extending to knee with tendency of bone pain and suppuration
- Tearing in the joint when sitting
- Cramp-like pain in the thumb joints
- Paralytic weakness of forearm
- Tremulous hands when using them
- Sensation in tips of fingers, as if suppurating

Symptoms *Worse*
- In the morning
- From washing
- From cold
- On uncovering the foot
- Lying down
- Drafts of air
- At night
- Lying on the left side
- Mental work
- Motion
- New moon
- Change of weather
- Getting wet

Symptoms *Better*
- Warmth (all symptoms except gastric one which are better by cold food)
- On wrapping the up head
- Summer

The following symptoms generally accompany the above symptoms . . .

- Useful in diseases of bones, caries and necrosis
- *Suppurative processes*, ripens abscesses since it promotes suppuration

- Ailment attended with *pus formation*
- Great sensitiveness to taking cold
- *Sensitive* to all impressions and *anxious*
- Headache better by *wrapping up warmly* and *when lying on the left side*
- Pain begins at back of head, and spreads all over head and settles over eyes
- *Profuse sweat of head*
- Tendency to inflammation, swelling and suppuration of glands—cervical, auxiliary, parotid, mamary. Small wounds heal with difficulty and suppurate easily
- *Pricking as if there is a pin in tonsil*
- Fissures and piles painful, with *spasm of sphincter of rectum*. Constipation, *stool* come down *with difficulty, when partly expelled, recedes again*
- *Night walking*—gets up while asleep
- Violent *cough* when lying down with *thick, yellow lumpy* expectoration
- White spots on nails
- *Promotes expulsion of foreign bodies* from tissues, e.g. thorn, splinters

Calcarea Carbonica 30

4 pills three times daily for one month

Symptoms

- It is a useful remedy for rheumatoid arthritis, chronic and acute muscular rheumatism, gouty nodosities
- Rheumatic pains, after getting wet
- Sharp sticking pain, as if parts were sprained

- *Cold, damp feet,* feels as if damp stocking were worn
- Pains are shooting, cutting or tearing, sometimes confined to small spots
- Pains are associated with cramps, contraction, stiffness and weakness all over the body
- Cold knees
- Cramp in calves
- Sour foot sweat
- Swelling of joints, especially knee
- Inflammation of hip joints which is painfully sore
- Burning of soles of feet which feel cold and dead at night
- Weakness in the muscles of thigh in morning, on beginning to walk, with stiffness, *worse while ascending stairs or any height*
- Pain in calves on stepping, on touch and on bending foot
- *Soles of feet raw*
- Ankles weary, feels as if dislocated
- Tearing in muscles
- Rheumatoid arthritis of finger joints with swelling and arthritic nodosities on hand and fingers joints

Symptoms *Worse*
- From excretion, mental or physical
- Ascending pain
- Cold in every form
- Washing, moist air, wet weather
- During full noon
- Standing
- After eating
- In the evening after midnight

Symptoms *Better*
- Dry climate and weather
- Lying on the painful side
- Sneezing
- Rubbing
- From drawing the limbs up
- While lying on the back in dark and dry weather

Bunions

- Pain in upper arm, as if beaten
- Sweating of palms of hands
- Sprained pain in right wrist, on motion
- Cramps in hands all night and trembling in the afternoon, worse from lifting heavy weights

The following symptoms generally accompany the above symptoms . . .

- It is generally suited to *children and women*
- The remedy is suited *to persons who are fatty, flabby and obese*
- Children whose head is too large, they *crave eggs and eat dirt,* and are prone to diarrhoea
- Children milestone are delayed especially while walking and talking
- There is great sensitiveness to catch cold
- *Profuse perspiration,* local and general, from slight exertion; *while sleeping wetting the pillow*
- Patient is very *apprehensive, forgetful* and has a variety of fears
- Sensation of coldness in general of single parts—head, stomach, feet and legs
- Periodicity of symptoms—commonly of 7 to 14 days
- *Enlarged glands*—Tonsils and other glands
- *Nostrils sore* and *ulcerated*
- Sour taste of mouth
- Craving of *indigestible things—chalk, coal, pencils*
- Frequent sour eructations, sour vomiting. *All discharges sour*
- Dislike of fat. May be aversion to milk
- *Loss of appetite when over worked*

- Menses *too early, too profuse, too long* with vertigo. *Milky white discharge*
- Painless hoarseness, shortness of breath on walking especially on going upstairs
- Aversion to open air
- Fever with night sweats, especially on head

Acid Benzoicum 30

4 pills three times daily for one month

Symptoms

- Useful in persons with *uric acid diathesis*
- It is a useful remedy in *gouty cases,* use it when *Colchicum* fails
- Swelling of the wrist with gout deposits
- Gouty deposits, nodes are very painful. Nodes on joints of fingers and toes
- Tearing pain in great toe
- *Bunion* of great toe
- Joint cracks on motion
- Tearing pain in tendons and joints with stitches
- *Pain in tendo-achilles*
- Pain and swelling in knees
- Oedema of the lower extremities
- Pain changes position suddenly, metastasise with heart pain in the cardiac region

Symptoms Worse
• In open air
• By uncovering
• Cold air
• Change in weather
• Motion
• Wine
• Urine scanty

Symptoms Better
• By heat
• Profuse urination

- ✦ Rheumatism and gout alternate with heart trouble with pain in the cardiac region

The following symptoms generally accompany the above symptoms . . .

- ✦ *Offensive odour* of urine accompanies the symptoms
- ✦ Urine is scanty, of a dark brown colour with repulsive odour; the smell exists at the time of urination and stays long afterwards
- ✦ Dribbling of urine in old men with enlarged prostate
- ✦ Renal insufficiency. Renal colic
- ✦ Rheumatism and gout alternate with heart trouble with palpitation and pain in cardiac region
- ✦ Stool offensive and liquid

Kali Iodide 30

4 pills three times daily for one month

Symptoms

- ✦ Rheumatic pain at night and in damp weather
- ✦ *Rheumatism of knee with effusion*
- ✦ Severe bone pains. Gnawing pain in left leg. Bones are sensitive to touch especially shin bone (leg bone)
- ✦ Contractions of joints
- ✦ Pain is hips causes limping when walking
- ✦ Gout affecting every joint with an indication that hepatic region is painful on touch

Symptoms *Worse*
- Warm clothing
- Warm room
- At night
- Damp, wet weather
- By touch
- At rest
- Lying on the painful side or on back

- Sensation as if small insects were crawling on the skin of lower extremities when sitting, better at lying down
- Rheumatism in *neck, back,* feet especially heels and soles gets worse with cold and wet

> **Symptoms *Better***
> - Open air (walking in open air, feels no fatigue)
> - Motion

The following symptoms generally accompany the above symptoms . . .

- It act prominently on fibrous and connective tissues, producing infiltration oedema
- *Glandular swelling*
- Emaciation and weakness
- Headache at *sides* and *root of nose*
- Profuse, *acrid, hot, watery, thin* discharge from nose
- Saliva increased, cold food and drink, especially milk, increases the suffering
- *Larynx feel raw.* Awakes choking. *Expectoration like soap-suds, greenish*
- Pimples with red tip

Rhododendron 30

4 pills three times daily for one month

Symptoms

- Well marked *rheumatic and gouty* symptoms
- It can affect *mainly small joints*
- Joints are red and swollen
- *Rheumatic tearing* in *all limbs,* especially on the right side
- Numbness and formication

- Rheumatic pain in bones in spots and reappear due to change of weather
- Pain in shoulders, arms and wrists
- Pain in limbs especially felt in the forearm and leg down to the fingers and toes
- Digging, drawing sprained pains in wrists
- Heaviness, weakness and tremors in hand
- Paralytic pain in right shoulder when resting open it, sometimes extending below elbow
- Heaviness in thighs. Pain in hips as if sprained
- *Cannot sleep unless legs are crossed*
- Gouty inflammation of great toe-joint with swelling and redness
- Acute and chronic gouty conditions

Symptoms *Worse*
- Before a storm
- All symptoms reappear in rough weather
- Windy weather
- Wet, cold weather
- At night
- Towards morning
- Rest
- Wine

The following symptoms generally accompany the above symptoms . . .
- Patient is gloomy, forgetful and afraid of thunderstorm
- All symptoms worse before a storm, relieved when it breaks
- Pain in lower jaw and chin, better from *warmth* and *eating*

Symptoms *Better*
- After a storm breaks
- Warmth
- Dry heat
- Exercise
- By eating
- From wrapping the head
- Immediately on starting to move

✦ Testicles intensely painful to touch, drawn up, swollen and painful. Hydrocoele

Sulphur 30
4 pills three times daily for fifteen days

Symptoms

✦ Rheumatic and arthritic complaints due to suppression of any skin disease
✦ *Painful stiffness* is main symptom, with or without effusion
✦ For preventing gouty diathesis there is no better remedy than *Sulphur*
✦ One of the leading remedy for synovitis
✦ *Hot, sweaty hands*
✦ Trembling of hands
✦ Sprained pain in wrist
✦ Pain in left shoulder as if joint is dislocated
✦ Jerking in deltoid
✦ Drawing pain in shoulder and arms
✦ Swelling in fingers in morning, sticking in tips at night; of flexure surface of right middle finger

Symptoms *Worse*
• At rest
• Around 11 a.m.
• In the morning
• At night
• Warmth of bed
• When standing
• Washing and bathing
• From alcoholic stimulants
• From weather changes
• Periodicity

Symptoms *Better*
• Dry, warm weather
• In open air
• Lying on the right side
• From drawing up affected limbs

- *Stoop shoulders*, cannot walk erect
- Tearing above the nail of left ring finger, worse in the evening
- Sharp draws, shooting and stitches here and there
- Pains seem to ascend, is worse in mid-summer heat, on clear and cloudless days
- Sweat in armpits, smelling like garlic
- Stiffness of knees and ankles
- *Burning in soles and hands at night*
- Weakness of thighs and legs
- Tearing extending into middle of the thigh, worse on standing and on ascending stairs
- Tearing through knee extending to feet when walking and sitting
- Sprained wrenching pain in joints with cracking and stiffness, particularly in knees and shoulders
- Sudden cramp-like, painful jerking about the hip joints with stiffness
- Tension, pain in joint on walking
- Tension in hollow of knees, as if too short, on stepping
- Inclination to cramp on stretching out feet
- Rheumatic gout with itching
- Swelling and inflammation of big toe with pain

The following symptoms generally accompany the above symptoms . . .

- Burning everywhere in the body especially head, palm and sole
- *Dirty, filthy people,* prone to skin disease, dry and hard hair and skin

- Children—*cannot bear to be washed or bathed*
- Aversion of being bathed
- *When carefully selected remedies fail to produce a favourable effect,* especially in acute disease
- Itching eruption on the skin. Scratching is followed by burning
- *Standing is the worse position* for patients, they cannot stand
- *Complaints are relapsing*—the patient seems to get almost well but the disease returns
- Redness of all orifices (lips, ears, eyelids, nostrils, anus, urethra etc.) as if pressed full of blood
- Discharges are offensive in character
- The discharges both of urine and faeces is painful to parts over which it passes; *parts around anus red, excoriated.* All the orifices of the body are very red
- Milk disagrees, craves sugar, sweets and tatty food
- *Great acidity* and sour eructations
- *Diarrhoea,* painless, *driving out of bed early in the morning*
- Weak, empty gone feeling and faints about 11 a.m.

Following an analysis of overall situation you can take remedies that may relieve pain and other symptoms. If there is no improvement after taking remedies then please consult a trained homoeopathic practitioner.

Home Remedies

- A heated pad or warm foot bath will relieve pain and discomfort

- Buy new comfortable shoes in place of an old one, to take pressure off a bunion

Prevention

Because bunions develop slowly, taking precautions as your feet grow can pay off later in life
- If foot problems run in your family, closely observe the shape of your feet
- Avoid shoes that cause cramps or pinch your toes
- Wear shoes that fit properly
- Women should be wary of high-heeled, pointed shoes styled more for fashion than for comfort and good support